An Ordinary Life

An Ordinary Life

Charles J. Alaimo

iUniverse, Inc.
New York Lincoln Shanghai

An Ordinary Life

Copyright © 2006 by Charles J. Alaimo

iUniverse books may be ordered through booksellers or by contacting:

iUniverse
2021 Pine Lake Road, Suite 100
Lincoln, NE 68512
www.iuniverse.com
1-800-Authors (1-800-288-4677)

ISBN-13: 978-0-595-38620-8 (pbk)
ISBN-13: 978-0-595-83000-8 (ebk)
ISBN-10: 0-595-38620-2 (pbk)
ISBN-10: 0-595-83000-5 (ebk)

Printed in the United States of America

For Gabriella and Anthony

Contents

Introduction

My Italian grandmother saved my childhood. A powerful influence during my youth, the memory of her is my rock in adulthood. Her very ordinary upbringing made my lonely, tortured childhood an extraordinary journey. Along the way I found love and courage, and learned to deal with the forces of my anxieties.

She accompanied me during the ordinary moments of family life—Sunday coffee in the backyard, holiday gatherings in the kitchen, chatting on the back stoop. The impact of these ordinary moments was compounded when in 1980 we learned of her cancer.

How often upon the passing of a loved one do we hear, "I wish I had spent more time with so and so," or "I wish we had traveled to such and such a place?"

It's easy for us to understand how the speed of life overrides such wishes. However, around us each day are moments we don't need to seek out, moments so ordinary we take for granted. I say enjoy them. Relish them. Blaze those moments into your mind.

My expectation for the readers of *An Ordinary Life* is for this book to heighten appreciation for every moment spent with loved ones. For readers currently living through the illness of a loved one, my story may be seen as a guide to sharing simple, ordinary events that can change the course of lives.

Prologue

There was little relief from the heat along the sun-baked roads of Castrofilippo that twenty-eighth day of September 1920, though every now and then a breeze whipped the ochre-colored dirt of Via Vittorio Emmanuele. Swirls of sand gently caressed the doorways and stone walls of homes lining the road. Behind one of the hand-hewn doors in this small Sicilian town with a population that hovered just around three thousand, a baby was about to be born to Diego Cinquemani and his wife, Concetta.

Concetta was twenty-five, relatively old by the standards of the time for birthing her first child. Diego was thirty-three. They had met in America, having emigrated from Italy like more than two million of their compatriots bound for America between 1900 and 1910.

Diego had departed Palermo, Sicily, on April 14, 1906 aboard the Austro-Americana Line's, *Gerty*. After eighteen days crossing the Atlantic, the three hundred and forty-six foot craft entered New York harbor on May second. With sixteen dollars to his name, nineteen-year-old Diego cleared immigration at Ellis Island dressed in a gray suit and went to live with a cousin of the same name who resided on Thirty-eighth Street in Manhattan.

The journey for seventeen-year-old Concetta Sedita was from the same point of departure and she also entered through Ellis Island, but that's where the similarity ended. On her first and only documented trip to America, her fifty-five year old father, Calogero accompanied her aboard the *Principe di Piemonte*. They had left her mother, Maria Messina in the one story stone structure they called home back in Castrofilippo, and had come to America to see Giuseppe, Concetta's brother, who resided on West Forty-sixth Street in Manhattan.

It's unclear how or when Diego and Concetta's paths crossed, but they were married in New York City in 1919 and returned to Sicily soon after.

◆　　◆　　◆

Before the afternoon was over, the Cinquemani's welcomed their first born, Maria, into the world. Her birth into this poor family was not marked by fanfare.

There were no birth announcements or a warm and snug cradle in which to place the infant, only a small drawer lined with coarse blankets to keep her warm during the cold evenings. Much like the local merchants who traveled ten miles a day leading mules carrying nut harvests over windy barren roads, Maria's life was to be a difficult journey.

Like most in the impoverished village twenty-five kilometers northeast of Agrigento, she was born into a family who relied on the sustenance of the earth for their livelihood. Her life was anything but idyllic, and was often difficult and sometimes tragic. There was no glamour in Maria's life, only hard lessons learned. No lavish events, no dressing up for parties, only tough, laborious work.

At the early age of four, Maria lost her mother. Fate was kind to her though, allowing the death at a time when she would not remember the sound of her mother's voice or the soft touch of her hand as she caressed Maria's face while she slept in the hay-stuffed bed. With a young child at home and the need to work, Diego soon remarried, thus ensuring he would have someone to take care of him and his young daughter.

Maria and her stepmother, Rosalia did not have the best of relationships compounded by the fact that Rosalia had children of her own—Salvatore, Concettina, and Antonia.

Although Maria grew up without the motherly love and affection, she had the support of her stepsiblings, who throughout her life were always very close and loving. One would never have known they were anything but brothers and sisters.

The years passed, and it wasn't long before teenage Maria caught the eye of Calogero Alaimo. Calogero, which means Charles in the southern Sicilian dialect, was a dreamer. He was a laborer who worked magic on his father's land turning the parched earth into a fertile oasis of grapes and squash. Much to his father's intense displeasure, Calogero dreamt of a better life in America.

Calogero's father Antonio, like most men of his time, had made the voyage to America many times to make money, in his case by gambling, and then returning home. On one of his trips to America in 1912, Antonio was joined by his wife Giuseppa Ciccotto.

After disembarking from the ship *San Giorgio* the thirteenth day of October, Giuseppa joined her husband in a small apartment at 661 First Avenue. Nine months later Calogero was born; a citizen of the United States. There was probably nothing he remembered about the United States since he returned to Sicily at the age of three months.

There is little doubt that the strapping and tall Charles was greatly influenced by his father's tales of life in America. Or perhaps he carried his citizenship as an American in his heart. He voiced his desire to go to America to his father who was anything but receptive.

Antonio, was an unforgiving man and thought only of the precedent that would be set if he allowed his son Calogero to leave their land. Surely he thought his other sons would follow suit. However, Charles' mind was made up and Antonio disinherited his son.

Upon Charles and Maria's nuptials in 1940, Antonio gave nothing to the new couple in terms of land to farm, as was customary in those days. Like the hands of Briscola he played in the bars he frequented, Antonio felt he had the upper hand to seal their fate. He held the one thing that was life and power to them—the land. He failed. With a family that grew and a war that called him into service, Charles never lost sight of his goal to go to America.

In early 1959, Charles headed to America alone. Soon after, he called for the rest of his family to join him and he booked passage for them on board the *Saturnia*.

In July 1959, his family sailed from Palermo's harbor. Maria, thirty-six at the time, was leaving the only homeland she had ever known. With their three children Antonio, Diego and Josephine in tow, she began her journey to America seeking the dream of so many—a better life. By all accounts they achieved their goal. Their three children went on to have families of their own, giving Maria and Charles several grandchildren.

I was the eldest.

1

Secrets and Loneliness

"Why is it that something always happens when I am away?" I thought to myself. The rush of wind coming in from the window of the sedan whipped my hair against my high forehead. "I hate my forehead," I thought without hesitation as another piece of hair whipped my right eye. It was too wide. That's why I kept the front of my hair longer than I really wanted it.

Perhaps equally as puzzling was the second question I asked myself. "Why is it that my family keeps things from me and only tells me things after I ask?" These two questions occupied my mind as the cab sped to O'Hare along the empty roads of an early Sunday morning.

I had arrived in the Windy City two days earlier after finding out about my grandfather's condition from my wife, Lisa. My parents knew his condition when I left New York on Friday morning, but failed to tell me for fear I would cancel my attendance at a management meeting. After I had hung up the phone with Lisa, I immediately called my mother to verify the information. Her response was as expected. "We didn't tell you because we didn't want you to cancel your trip." It was terribly considerate of them. The only consolation was I would only be away two days.

Resting my chin on the knuckles of my left fist, I gazed out the window, my eyes fixated on, but not really paying attention to the airport train running parallel to my yellow taxi sedan. Having given myself plenty of time before my Delta flight back to New York, I quietly relished the fact that I would be able to spend some time browsing the airport gift shops, and more exciting to me, having time to sip a cup of coffee while viewing the planes on the tarmac. The cab turned with a jerk. I was sent nose first toward the finger-smudged window. I quickly caught a glimpse of myself in the glass pane. My forehead wrinkled as I squinted back at my reflection. My goateed face gave too harsh an impression when compared to the person inside.

The cab turned up the ramp to the departure area. I had finally arrived at the sunlit terminal. I slid across the navy vinyl upholstery choosing to get out on the side that faced the curb rather than into traffic. The cool air greeted me as I opened the door.

"Can I have a receipt?" I asked the driver before stepping out of the vehicle. The sound of my own voice seemed foreign to me. It felt good to stand and I took the opportunity to stretch my legs. Standing on the toes of my brown lace-ups, I inhaled deeply. I quickly adjusted my cropped leather jacket before grabbing my gray mesh companion, my favorite luggage that had quietly kept me company in the backseat. The wheels on one end of the case hit the sidewalk just as the driver walked to where I was standing. I gave him the fare plus a generous tip, usual for me, and the driver handed over the receipt, his fingers bent as if still wrapped around the steering wheel. I guess he must have been driving a car for a good part of his life. The large bones of his knuckles were highlighted by deep crevices of white, dead, flaky skin. I gently folded the receipt and placed it in the inner pocket of my waist-length black coat.

"Thank you," I said warmly.

He nodded. "Safe trip." His gray hair waved in a light breeze wafting from the upper level of the terminal. He made his way back to his seat and with a slam of the door was off to grab his next passenger. I stood on the curb a few seconds watching him drive away. Nicholas (I had extrapolated the driver's name from the license hanging on the front dashboard) seemed like a nice older gentleman, and I felt bad for not having been more of a conversationalist during our forty minutes together.

An increasing sense of loneliness enveloped me. Here was another person who had entered my life and just as quickly, exited. How easy it was for someone to come into your life and then leave. Had I learned anything about this guy during our ride? Did I get a sense of who he was?

I continued to stand there looking down the crowded concourse, my cab long gone. I felt unable to move until the wonderfully loud sound of a jetliner climbing toward the cobalt blue sky saved me from my thoughts.

"A 777," I muttered as my eyes caught the bright flash of the sun streaking across the wing of this brand new silvery bird.

Over the past year, I was reacquainted with my love of planes and airports. As early as I could recall, I had always been fascinated with planes. I looked up and saw the triple seven climb into a white fluffy cloud and out of view. I took another deep breath and allowed the unique airport scent, a mix of catered food and jet fuel, to infiltrate my senses. I grabbed my bag and headed into the coolness and safety of the building.

After an exhausting visit to almost every store in the accessible area of the terminal, I finally made my way to the gate. I had to go through the metal detector twice (my big silver belt buckle the culprit) and endure a search with a metal wand.

A round, uniformed guard gabbed amusingly with her seated co-worker about her supervisor giving her early shifts two days in a row. Her highlighted curly hair fell lightly against her smooth cheeks. She had a fun air of attitude about her.

"What's he thinkin', like I ain't got no life?" She kept the wand hovering around my belt buckle and other private areas.

"I should just hit him upside the head," she laughed in a throaty rasp. She looked at her friend for validation but found none. Her co-worker was as indifferent to her chatter as to the x-ray screen she viewed. Not getting a response, the plump woman switched her gaze to me. My arms were still outstretched. I smiled along with her and she liked that.

"You can go, sweetheart," she gave me a tap on the side of my leather coat.

"If it's any consolation, what you're going through happens to all of us," I said as I gathered my bag now buried under two sweaters and a beige purse at the end of the conveyor belt.

She smiled.

I quickly looked at her badge. "Have a good one, Gloria." I parted some last words of advice over my shoulder. "Don't let it get to you."

I turned to look back; Gloria continued looking my way as I dragged my friend behind me. Having worked in the service industry for many years, and having been employed by a few airlines, I was almost instantaneously drawn to name badges or IDs. It was part of the training in the service sector to use a person's name no less than three times in a conversation. But I didn't need to be taught this, it was something ingrained in me even before I started working.

I had always been sensitive and mindful of others. I use names to enter into conversation, albeit briefly, which probably dissipated from memory two seconds later for the other person, but not me. I relished these encounters, the chance to meet people in different situations, in different parts of the country. People I would not ordinarily meet exhilarated me, temporarily filling my huge need, or want, or gap. Whatever it might be called it had existed for most of my life; this need to be wanted, to feel important, and to be supported. Not only to be a friend, but to have friends. I wanted serious conversation on the meaning of current experiences in my life. The frustration, the boredom, the loneliness, the despair, the depression, the worthlessness. I did a pretty good job hiding it all.

Bag in tow, I walked the long finger of the gate area, my youthful face of thirty-three years turned upward. My brown eyes, hazel green after a good cry, searched for L5 in a sea of brown and white signs, some with symbols for telephones or restrooms. Every now and then my gaze wandered to the multitude of flagpoles adorning the length of the arched glass terminal.

Within a few minutes I found my gate. I had hit the jackpot! Gate L5 offered sweeping views of the tarmac and the jetway before me still awaited an aircraft. My eyes searched again, this time for a place to sit. I proceeded to the row of chairs closest to the windows. A bit of loose carpet caused me to stub the right toe of my shoe causing a slight trip in my usual brisk and sure stride.

I plopped on the seat, one in a row of six, like a sack of laundry, my brown hair slapping across my forehead and into my eyes. I had purchased a large cup of coffee. I placed it on the seat beside me and grabbed my wheeled traveling companion and propped it beneath my legs like a footstool. It was nirvana to allow my legs to rest on the densely packed piece of luggage. Reaching for the hot brew, I lifted the white and green cup to my mouth and took a long slow sip of no-whip mocha, and with hidden glee and sheer delight I enjoyed the vista of arriving and departing aircraft. My mind wandered. A not unusual occurrence these days. I often get lost in thought or some other amusement—like listening through blaring headphones to a favorite CD.

This time, however, my distractions were thoughts of the few and far between happy moments of my childhood. I say that because my worries then equaled my worries now.

◆　　　◆　　　◆

Charles often made the trip to visit Nonna alone.

Charles always called his grandmother Nonna.

The walk alone was fine for him since it was only around the block or four hundred and ten paces.

He had counted.

Today however, Charles was not alone. His mom tagged along to learn some new sewing stitches from her well-versed mother-in-law. In addition, a brand new unopened model airplane kit also accompanied the tall and lanky youngster. Still wrapped in its crispy cellophane wrapper, the box rustled from underneath his armpit.

He walked with great strides, a result borne out of necessity to keep up with his father. His gym socks fell just shy of his large, bony kneecaps. The red and orange horizontal stripes on the socks matched his red gym shorts and gray tank. His belly shook as he walked.

The cool air invigorated him causing him to lose track of his steps around two hundred and thirty while he walked under the train overpass running perpendicular to the block.

Charles was a good twenty feet ahead of his mom as he climbed the stairs leading to the front door. He rang the bell to his grandparent's modest two-story row house and waited for the door to open.

He stood on the tips of his toes to peer through the lowest window on the door. His hands rested on the brick façade of the house as he tried to look inside.

His grandmother, Maria, emerged from the living room to the left of the hallway. Her gaze caught her grandson's. She gave a great big smile. He heard the door unlock. She was still smiling as she threw open the storm door.

At ten years of age, Charles was already six feet tall and stood six inches taller than Maria. "Hi, Nonna." Charles stooped down to kiss her. He was truly happy to see her.

"Ciali," she said in her broken Sicilian accent. She kissed her grandson's right cheek and slapped the other cheek with affection.

No matter the day, the week or the month, and no matter how often they stood together on the threshold of the hallway lined with beautiful and verdant plants in equally beautiful jardinières, they were always happy to see one another.

Her eyes were dark and pensive and always genuine. They mirrored the soul of this ordinary grandmother and simple lady who emitted nothing but love.

Charles hugged her and went into the house. Nonna turned to welcome her daughter-in-law who by now had made it up the brick steps. Charles walked a few steps down the hallway that bridged the entrance with the backyard door in the small kitchen.

"Barbara, how…"

Charles disappeared through the doorway to his right. His sneakers carried him down the brown-treaded staircase that landed on the faux-marble tiles of the immaculately kept sub room.

Charles had spent much of his young life in this two-story, attached brick house, and close to sixty percent of that time in the basement. To him, however, it was more than just a basement. With its open floor plan and loads of natural light from the large windows and door leading to five large steps up to the backyard, the basement was a gathering place for those everyday dinners.

It was a place where Nonna made her homemade pasta on the large dining table in the center of the room. It was a place to watch television, and a place where all the holiday meal prep work began. It was home.

With the sunlight beaming in, Charles picked a place on the floor close to the far end of the room. Before sitting down, he pulled out a tube of model glue from the pocket of his shorts. The basement floor was damp and cold against the bareness of his legs, but that soon disappeared as he got into the act of building the latest addition to his growing collection of passenger planes; a TWA 727.

After gluing the newest model, painting the wings bright silver and applying the signature red and white decals, Charles proceeded to fly it all the way home.

◆   ◆   ◆

I was still laughing at the thought of having flown that handmade jet home in the grasp of my forefinger and thumb replete with my perfected sound effects, when I noticed an aircraft approaching the window. The massive structure of white with blue and red stripes across its nose and down the length of the fuselage came to a halt alongside the jetway. This was my favorite plane, the Boeing 767. In high school and even earlier on, I had thoughts of becoming a pilot. But that went out the door when I realized I needed to take classes in physics, mathematics, science, etc. So I just settled for being a passenger, and for the most part, I enjoy that role tremendously.

The ache in the inner core of my body was back. I closed my eyes. It was the ache I knew all too well and one that always tagged along on these trips. I took a deep sigh and opened my eyes to find a young couple sitting to my right holding hands. The woman's head leaned on her companion's shoulders. Her wavy brown hair covered his face as he no doubt inhaled the sweet smell of her shiny chestnut mane.

I sighed and smiled, not realizing which one I had done first. I understood why I had sighed. Simply put, I could not relate to how they were feeling. It had been a long time since I had felt like that, of being totally understood and supported. As for the smile, it was probably to hide the fact that my rear had fallen asleep from sitting on the hard, blue plastic chair.

I sat upright and moved gingerly to avoid the pins and needles feeling now spreading from my buttocks down my left leg. I leaned forward and stretched, and then placed my elbows just above my knees creasing my beige khakis. My shoulders felt heavy with tension and stress. As I glanced down at the scuffed industrial grade, gray carpet, I couldn't help but wonder why the designers of these terminals didn't make these waiting chairs with high backs. These low seats were horrible for anyone's neck. But yet I wasn't sure if I should place all the blame on the chairs. I just did not have the energy to go through another family member's illness again. The sheer selfishness of that thought made me question myself. But it was true.

There was no getting around the fact that I was drained; burnt out by the rigors of my job, a personal life that at best I barely maintained, and now I must face the fact my grandfather was dying. This was the proverbial last straw. I wanted to just stop what I was doing and spend as much time as I could with my grandfather.

Still leaning forward, wisps of hair covered my eyes and obstructed my trance-like view of the activity going on just beyond the window and all around me. I wished I had spent more time with Nonno, my grandfather. I wished I had acted on those spur of the moment whims to just pop by his house and say hello. What made me feel even worse was recalling the times when Nonno often asked me to stop by and visit.

My grandfather had to know the feelings I had toward him were much less than those for my grandmother. I felt guilty about this. The responsibilities of life, work, and children got in the way. As his time was coming to a close, I was, it seemed, far from that inevitable destiny.

"Ladies and gentlemen, in a few short moments—" the boarding call had begun. The jovial clerk went on, her voice optimistic and upbeat. "We ask that any passengers traveling with infants and—"

I was all too familiar with the boarding ritual. It was amazing how everyone seemed to rush up to the line even though the boarding began with the last five rows. Judging from the line today, it seemed like a good two-thirds of the plane was sitting in rows thirty-five to forty-one, no doubt a bit tail heavy.

I took my time. The luxury of traveling Business Class calmed my nerves and allowed me to board at my leisure. I also did not have to fight for space in the overheads once on board.

I stood in line. After the few parents and their children, along with strollers and the like were on board, Business Class began. I glanced to the couple who had caught my eye earlier. They were oblivious to the long line forming for their flight. The same agent who made the boarding call (Victoria, her nameplate read), took my ticket and fed it through the computerized gate gadget.

"Have a pleasant flight," she smiled, and handed me my stub. With that, I was on my way.

A little 'hurrah' went off in my stomach as I walked down the sparsely filled jetway. Soon I would be in the warm embrace of my Business Elite seat where I would be able to stretch out and relax and enjoy the luxury of the ample space. The free drinks didn't hurt either. Fear was not even a factor for me. Flying was second nature and provided me the 'rush' I needed to feel alive. In the event that something ever happened, I knew my family would be well taken care of financially with my various life insurance policies.

My footsteps echoed on the floor of the carpeted, white-walled jetway lined with pictures of places I wanted to see—Rio de Janeiro, Frankfurt, and Vienna. I loved international travel. The sound of my steps sounded as bleak and hollow as I felt inside. I was lonely and had been for some time. Once again a trip was coming to an end and I had nobody to return to. There was nobody to chat with or share the experiences of my journey. A journey that would never be repeated. Oh sure, I would probably go back to Chicago someday, but it would be different. It wouldn't be like this trip.

I reached the aircraft door and handed my boarding card to the older of two flight attendants greeting passengers. With her hair pulled back and a slight accent (Hungarian, I thought), she gave the impression of the past elegance of air travel. At the same time, I followed my boarding ritual, which was to tap on the fuselage of the aircraft upon entering. Today, my right fingers gently tapped on the fuselage of the shiny white bird bedecked in Delta's new colors. "Get me there safe, big bird," I muttered under my breath. This little saying was the final part of the rite.

Having entered the cabin, I found 3A, a window seat. Since I had been told there was nobody sitting on the aisle, I threw my carryon on next to me and stretched before sitting. The cabin's blue and gray colors warmed me. I felt at ease on this aircraft. The cozy seat embraced me. The leather relaxed me. I looked out the window to the blue sky above.

"Thank goodness it's a clear day," I thought to myself.

Sitting up front was enjoyable and luxurious, but did very little to build my self-esteem. I tried not to make eye contact with the many passengers passing through the Business Class cabin on their way to the back of the plane.

"Jill, look at these seats!" an older woman said to her traveling companion.

"Right nice, Ma," the woman replied. The daughter gently laid her fingers on the old woman's white knitted sweater and pushed her mother along. Then there were those who just looked at the wide cabin, the seats with five feet of generous legroom, and then looked at those sitting in the main cabin. A mix of jealousy and envy and a bit of wonderment crossing their faces. I surmised they probably thought to themselves, "What do these people do for a living that they are able to fly like this?" Although it may have seemed to the masses that I had 'arrived,' internally I felt anything but.

Similar to the coach passengers who passed me by, I looked to my comrades in the front cabin with the same wonderment and questioned how they were able to afford to sit up front. I could always make out the businessman or woman whose company was footing the bill.

"Surely to fly in Business Class they must be someone," I thought as I concurrently questioned my stature in belonging to such a group. I wanted my wife to experience this luxury. To acknowledge that in some way I had made it. I wanted her validation. But ever since Gabriella, our firstborn came into the world, Lisa had become terrified of flying. It seemed like yesterday the both of us were jetting off to someplace new, sharing the experience together. These days the experience was mine and mine alone. Even after my frequent trips were over, Lisa often did not want to hear about them. She hated when I had to travel. I gathered it wasn't because of a fear of anything happening to me, but about the inconvenience it caused her.

I could think of several things that would place me in such unfavorable light, like drinking shamelessly, having a clandestine affair (none of which I was guilty, mind you). But to be made to feel guilty for doing my job and supporting my family wasn't one of them.

So besides the fact that I had to travel alone, I was also saddled with a huge burden of guilt, which was slowly taking its toll. After giving and giving for so many years, all I wanted and needed was to have someone there for me, to give me the same support and understanding I had dispensed to so many. Basically, I needed a friend like myself to be there for me.

To a large degree, the career path I had chosen for myself twelve years earlier also placed me in the unique position of the giver. A human resources professional by trade, people are always approaching me for advice, for help on their issues. Even if I were not in this role, my demeanor was perfect for it.

One former boss even referred to me as the 'Confessor.' There's something about me that make people comfortable. I possess an approachable demeanor combined with a genuine nature to want to help and to keep confidences. This was ingrained and inherent in me. It was one of the traits that made me vulnerable to attack and subject to my own emotions, which at times got the best of me.

There was so much personal reward in my role, but all the giving went unreplenished. You could say I was a bank. People came from all over to make withdrawals, but no one ever made deposits. If this continued, the bank would eventually run dry. That is where I was at this point. Dry and thirsty for support and love.

I often wondered how ironic it was that internally I battled all my demons while being the source of advice and sound counsel to so many. The façade I had created of being unflappable in the midst of chaos worked. My own sense of self-worth was nil despite all the good in my life. At my core I was unhappy.

One of my flaws, if you call it that, was my need to always have something going on in my life, something to look forward to. That 'something' could have been a business trip, any trip, or a party perhaps.

My love of airplanes had more to do with how they paralleled my thoughts and feelings rather than their sheer beauty and power. They were always moving forward, climbing, the world laid out before them. My ambition, my need to succeed, was the fuel that pushed me forward climbing higher and faster. My goals yet to be achieved were before me, but at times I was unable to see through the clouds and turbulence of my life to get a clear picture of what exactly those goals were. With so much converging in my life, it wasn't even clear what I wanted on a daily basis, let alone a few years ahead.

2

Another Summer, Another Death

The warmth of the August afternoon sun shining through the train window felt good against my face. The view of the outside world was distorted by the etching of someone's name in the Plexiglas pane. No doubt the vandal's name or gang 'tag.' The train rolled slowly along and then halted suddenly between stations. Gazing through the carved pane from my vantage point high above the tracks, I stared into the offices of a small two-story building, one of many that lined the avenue.

Two very different scenes played out before me. In one office a dentist, clearly recognizable from his green garb, chatted with a patient. In the other an attorney (at least that's what I thought), fumbled through paperwork in his overstuffed leather chair. On the walls of both offices hung framed diplomas and certificates. Each man oblivious to the other proceeded simultaneously with their routine, their offices and lives separated by a wall.

I sighed just as the train jerked forward and rumbled back to life. Had it not been for my quick reflexes—grabbing onto the metal pole with my right hand—I would have body-slammed the elderly and quite smelly man beside me.

Having been home in New York for a day now, I was on my way to the hospital to visit my grandfather. It was the right thing to do. But as was always the case with me, everything involved much thought and self-discussion. Just a few minutes earlier I had debated whether or not to go. I knew the answer was obvious. Of course I had to go. What choice did I have?

My father, on the other hand, understood more than me, his eldest son. "You have a family. There's nothing you can do for your grandfather," he told me in a cell phone conversation. "Just go home and be with your family."

I made my way to the other side of the train. Standing at the doorway with one stop to go, I made sure I was one of the first to get off. Nobody was going to

beat me. My quiet demeanor hid the competitor deep inside. Even the most trivial things such as being the first to get off a train became a competition. I was
surely not about to let the well-dressed suit ahead of me win. My khakis were
more casual than my fellow traveler's dark pin stripes, and instead of a leather
briefcase I opted for a gray messenger bag. Little did the stranger know that I
probably earned more money in one year than he in two, but there was little I
could do to announce this fact. "And besides," I thought, "who wears a blue suit
in August?" I internally mocked my fellow traveling companion.

The train came to an abrupt stop and I flew off down the stairs almost missing
a step as my legs moved faster and faster as if they had a mind of their own. While
running down the two flights to the street, I took out my black cell phone. I
dialed as I walked making sure to look up every now and then so I did not bump
into the throngs of people. I needed to tell my parents of my decision to go to the
hospital, and I wanted to make sure my wife had dinner at their house.

"Hello?" Lucky for me my wife Lisa answered.

I responded to her question as to my whereabouts. "I'm on my way to the hospital now. I just got off the train. Why?" She already sounded pissed that she had
to wait for me to get home. I walked fast and spoke even faster as I strode along
Thirtieth Avenue or Grand Avenue as it was referred.

I passed store windows catching reflections of myself in the glass. The stores
and people made this area so diverse, very different from what I remembered
growing up there so many years ago when the area was predominantly Italian.

I dodged the slow moving pedestrians as if they were orange traffic cones in
the road. Living in the gentrified suburbs of Long Island for the past five years, I
felt out of my element walking these streets, feeling almost uncomfortable. For
the longest time after we had moved into our saltbox colonial, replete with green
lawn and white picket fence, coming into Queens to drop off my daughter at my
parents was a harsh reality for me. It seemed like everyone lived on top of one
another, like a heap of laundry where everything was mixed together. I missed the
diversity.

The day was warm. Beads of sweat formed on my forehead. I could feel drips
running from my armpits and down my torso.

Lowering my voice into a deep, hushed whisper, I wrapped up the conversation with my wife. "Hey, I've got to go. I'm about to enter the hospital and they
don't like these cell phones on."

My throat burned after that four-block walk. "Okay, I'll see you at home
soon," I said.

My head began to ache from squinting, thanks to the late afternoon sun in my eyes during the walk from the train station to the big brick hospital building. Scaffolding outside the entranceway provided much-needed shade allowing my eyes to readjust.

"Okay, bye Lee," I said impatiently. I looked down at my watch. I had to bring the dial close to my face to make out the hands hidden from view by the bright sun.

"Don't worry, we'll discuss it later, bye," I said again, trying once and for all to end the conversation. "Right. Fine. Bye." Lisa was trying to decide if she should take a vacation day from work tomorrow. It was the last thing I wanted to discuss at that moment.

I snapped the palm-sized phone closed. Like a tortoise shell, the thin plastic cover converted into a compact little object. I threw the phone into my shoulder bag. The gray mesh strap creased my neck. I quickly repositioned it around my shoulder and hurried past the waiting lounge and the security desk (if that's what you want to call it) then to the elevators.

"Ahh," I sighed thinking to myself in front of the elevator door. "It's nice to see some things never change, like these pathetically slow elevators."

Pacing back and forth, I caught bits of conversation from the shuffling humanity who made their way to and from the Emergency Room just around the corner. The smell of antiseptic filled the low ceiling corridor. Oh, how I hated hospitals, and in particular this one. Perhaps because my grandmother had died here or possibly because compared to hospitals in Manhattan, this place reminded me of something impermanent and makeshift.

The mauve walls and highly-glossed floors hadn't changed in all the years I had visited. I grew dizzy from scanning the black and white tiled floors that formed a complex harlequin pattern.

"They say she needs surgery to remove…" one stout man said to his much younger companion. "They give her only a few months," said another passerby. I managed to hear pieces of life and death discussions. Another woman walked by to my right walking arm in arm with a young girl. The woman's lips moved, but the conversation was too low to be overheard.

My eyes veered to one part of this long passageway. A small corner I knew all too well, a significant place. A doctor stood there now, or at least I thought it was a doctor.

My gaze fixated on that corner spot where nineteen years ago I was part of a scene similar to those that were now playing out around me.

◆   ◆   ◆

Nonna had been in excruciating pain. At her doctor's request, the family admitted her to the hospital. She walked in with her eldest grandson Charles supporting her on one side, and her son Tony on the other. Luckily, a wheelchair was available and they gently placed her in it.

Charles had grown accustomed to carefully lifting her legs out of the way before swinging down the metal footrests of the wheelchair.

All the while she cried. "Ai! Ai!"

Nonna couldn't move her legs on her own. She needed someone to maneuver them for her. When Charles accompanied her to the many doctor's appointments, he always put her in the passenger side of his aunt's car. He supported most of Nonna's weight by placing his left arm underneath her shoulders. He placed her gently on the seat, knelt to clasp her legs together, and then carefully placed her feet on the floor.

Nonna helped too, shifting her weight and direction with her arms. She held one arm against the seat, the other on the car's middle console. It was a synchronized task.

Charles' grandmother had lost most of her sense of taste, a result of the bombardment from chemo and cobalt treatments. As was the case today, she often carried a nice Bartlett pear in a paper napkin that she occasionally bit into when the pain became increasingly intolerable.

If she was fortunate, there was a long span between bites.

By the time she unwrapped the pear the second or third time, the edges where she had last bitten had already turned brown.

Charles could not begin to fathom the pain his grandmother was experiencing. The cancer at this point was terminal and had affected her legs. She spent an enormous amount of time in bed, and this brought a whole new set of problems like painful bed-sores.

Charles' attempts to console his grandmother had no effect. He felt powerless to help her.

Her cries increased as his father lifted Nonna from the wheelchair by placing his arms under her legs while she clutched his neck.

Her tan sleeveless dress, which she had made herself, enveloped her. Her eldest son placed her gently on an unoccupied stretcher in the corner of the hallway. Charles looked on, standing with his hands deep in the pockets of his baggy jeans. The picture of his dad helping his mother was emblazoned in his mind forever.

"Ai!" she sobbed while taking a deep breath.

She lay on her left side propped up by her arm, her back to the wall.

"Ai!" she cried again.

With every cry she gritted her teeth. Her cheeks pulled up around her eyes as she grimaced. Her body writhed on the white-sheeted stretcher as the intense pain pierced through her small five foot three-inch frame.

Charles continued to look, but did not say a word. His face said it all. He leaned against the metal railing and looked at her face, too paralyzed to do much else.

Although Nonna was only about three weeks away from her sixtieth birthday, she had a young appearance. The hardships caused by her illness during the past year had only minimal effects on her visage.

As Charles, his father, and grandfather stood there in the middle of the hallway across from the cashier's window, they were unable to look at one another as they waited for word of a vacant room.

They were helpless to do anything more as her cries grew more intense.

◆   ◆   ◆

Pinngg. Pinngg.

My recollection was interrupted by the sound of the warped elevator signal. It had finally made its way down from the sixth floor. Shaking my head I could not even begin to understand how these elevators operated so slowly; especially in a building with only six floors. Inhaling and then exhaling deeply, I tried to release the aggravation that had built up from the wait. I wiped my eyes as I entered the six by seven foot car and scanned the worn, black keys looking for the fourth floor. My fingertips touched the smooth edges of the buttons, the white numbers barely visible from years of abuse by other frustrated individuals and families.

Just as I depressed the button, a small lady entered the elevator. I moved to the back of the car. She could barely keep her fingers from pumping the number two button.

"It's not going to move any quicker if you keep pressing the life out of it," I thought to myself, and wishing I could say it aloud. "In the time we waited for the doors to close, you could have climbed the two flights," I mumbled, and stamped my foot in aggravation. Only when I allowed my eyes to look down did I realize climbing wasn't even a possibility. Her legs were as wide as her hips and with her short frame I concluded that taking on the hospital's stairs would for her be like a trek up Machu Picchu.

I had been in the hospital for close to ten minutes and had still not seen the person I came to see. All this was a big waste of time.

Finally, I reached the fourth floor. This was the same floor my grandmother had spent her final days.

Room 409, I remembered. My forehead wrinkled as I tried hard to recall. It was on this same floor in a room down this same nondescript hallway with its sickening bland walls and pictures that seemed from some street corner vendor. Yes, I had indeed been here before, only the person in the bed was different.

I made a left turn at the nurse's station and walked a few more steps down a short corridor and came upon Room 426. I saw Nonno immediately. He occupied the first bed closest to the hallway. His eyes were open.

"Hi, Nonno," I said, as I entered the room and patted the silver railing on the bed.

There was no response.

"Nonno?" I leaned forward calling his name again a bit louder, but not too loud for the sake of his other two roommates blocked from my view by a fabric wall.

My grandfather continued to stare ahead, his eyes wide open, yet motionless. Not even a blink. He was sleeping. I made sure this was so by checking the rise and fall of his chest.

I touched the sheet. It was cold like the rest of the room, which was divided by soft flowing, pink-hued curtains that hung from steel rings on a steel track.

I took a seat on the wide chair next to the bed, moved my shoulder bag alongside me, and leaned against the thick wooden armrest. I would have been here sooner had I known how grave Nonno was. I thought again of how my parents did not share with me the severity of his condition. Granted, there wasn't much I could do, but I grew angrier as I realized how my mom and dad always skirted issues around me. I fidgeted in my seat.

There's no question that over the past few years I had become quite opinionated and vocal in my family. On several occasions my father would comment to others that he didn't know who his son took after.

On the surface my father and I were nothing alike. My tastes were extravagant, my father preferred simplicity. He felt material items only brought worry and clutter. I, on the other hand, held a firm belief that life should be lived, money would come and go. Dad's impoverished upbringing had left an indelible imprint on him, which governed the way he lived even though he had enough money for better things. Living off the land, as his family had done, brought little in the way of luxuries. Having meat once a week was about the only one.

Life was difficult for the family, and my dad Tony, being the eldest, was a mirror image of his mother. Many chores needed to be accomplished such as accompanying his father from town to town, an entire day's journey for them. Walking through the dusty roads from his village of Castrofilippo to the surrounding towns like Canicatti, all by foot, was no easy task. And all to sell nuts.

In times where food was scarce, my dad knew what it meant to be hungry. He knew the experience of losing a brother, who at the age of one, died from malnutrition. My dad had told me how his brother Diego (my grandmother had a subsequent son whom they named Diego, my uncle) was waked on the kitchen table. Hearing these stories from him, I understood where my dad was coming from.

Even now he would recycle old pieces of wood to make garden furniture. A wooden door became a bench. If he bought a pair of shoes with tassels, he ripped them off. Having the money now to afford things made him feel guilty in some way, at least that was my theory. So by doing these small things it reminded him of his humble upbringing in Sicily.

Although my father and I were different in many ways, we were very much alike inside; in our beliefs of family and religion, which were important. I wasn't quite sure if my father realized the similarities between us. My exterior was just a good front so not to appear weak.

And so here I sat in the muted sunlit room watching another grandparent die. The muffled din of life going on about the streets below provide some relief from the heavy silence in the room, interspersed with the occasional announcement over the PA system. Every now and then sounds of laughter drift down the hallway from the nurse's station.

I reach for the bed sheet. It is the closest thing I can touch without touching my grandfather. I cannot bring myself to laying a hand on my namesake's swollen arm. His flesh is tight and oozing water, much like a sausage whose outer casing is stretched to the limit. I realize it is probably infected from a combination of the IV, and that he had been retaining water since I last saw him two weeks ago. My family had gathered for a barbeque to celebrate his eighty-seventh birthday. Prior to that day, whenever I had asked my father how Nonno was doing, he always responded the same way. "He's doing fine, he looks good." I got the feeling this was a canned response because since December, Nonno had suffered with bouts of phlebitis.

My dad was convinced this was a result of his father taking a spill from a ladder while painting. "Yeah, sounded just like Nonno," I said, when I first heard the news. "Stubborn, that's what he is."

My grandfather was very headstrong and determined for as long back as I could recall. Yet, when I saw him that hot July day for his birthday celebration, I just couldn't believe he was the same man.

3

A Picnic in July, 2000

Dad emerged from the kitchen door. Its squeaky metal frame slammed shut as he came down the cement stairs to the yard. There was something about the painted gray steps that made me stop and think. So many of my relatives used that same battleship gray color to paint just about everything from basement walls to the cement in their backyard.

My father had returned from his walk around the block to get Nonno. Rather than come through the backyard entrance, he chose to go through the front door so Nonno could rest a bit in the living room. Nonno must not have been feeling well because he had left his motorized scooter at home. He and Martha, the woman he had married a few years after Nonna's death, had matching scooters but in different colors. They could often be seen maneuvering through the streets of Astoria after grocery shopping or just cruising along.

I walked past Dad on my way in to say hello to 'Charlie Number 1' as my grandfather sometimes referred to himself. I was of course 'Number 2.' As I made the slight right hand turn past the kitchen sink filled with dirty Corning Ware and a few utensils, I saw Nonno sitting on the sofa. His gray-buttoned sweater hung loose. His stare blank and his cheeks hollow. I could not believe this was my grandfather.

"Hi, Nonno." Sickened by his appearance, my cheekbone pressed against his as we kissed.

"Ciali." His response barely audible, my grandfather called my name.

His eyes were sunken, his face ashen and sallow. Nonno had been thin in recent years, but now he looked especially gaunt. His mouth remained opened, almost as if he wasn't able to close his jaw due to the muscles loosing their elasticity. The gray pants and sweater Nonno wore only made his complexion appear worse.

"Is this what my father thinks is looking good?" I said to myself.

I shook my head then exited the house and returned to the backyard.

"Da, he looks terrible. My God, I can't believe how much worse he looks," I said as I walked over to where my aunt, uncle and cousins were all sitting around the big wooden picnic table. I looked over to my aunt. Josephine had just taken a big bite of her barbequed hamburger that looked more like a meatball on a bun.

"He looks bad, Jo," I repeated.

She didn't look at me, but intently dabbed her burger with some additional ketchup. She shook her head back and forth, her straight black hair bobbing just above her shoulders. I think she knew I was right.

My father didn't say much as he took a seat at the picnic table. It was a table he had made himself. The white t-shirt he wore hung loose from his thin five-foot six-inch frame. For as long as I could recall, my father had never gained or lost an ounce.

My dad was in denial about just how sick Nonno was. I shouldn't have been surprised that my father's words did not validate the reality of Nonno's condition. He wanted his father to be well so he had conveniently overlooked his father's deteriorating condition.

By the time we were ready to eat, Dad had disappeared into the house to get Nonno. My grandfather was not able to walk for long periods without help, but often insisted on doing just that. Determined to remain independent, Nonno came down the stairs from the kitchen. As a precaution, my dad came right behind, his spectacled eyes watching Nonno's every move for any sign of falter. With each step, my grandfather's thin, bony legs protruded from the workman pants he always wore (again in a battleship gray color). He took his seat as was de rigueur at these backyard get-togethers beneath the natural shelter of Italian squash leaves and grape vines.

Nonno and my father took great pleasure in gardening. In the late spring, each could be found tilling the soil. My grandfather, at almost six feet, was adept at maneuvering his long thin legs over the piles of dirt he pushed toward him to make graceful mounds, which separated the beds. He and my father spent a lot of time together getting the ground ready to plant while chatting about whatever it was they chatted about.

By this time of the summer, the awning overhead and the plants in the garden should have been lush and green. My father and Nonno grew figs, grapes and *gugutsa*, the long Italian squash that resembled baseball bats. There should have been at least ten gugutsa hanging from the vine by now with everyone dodging them as they walked underneath the awning. For some reason, this year everything looked bare.

Patches of sky were visible through the natural canopy and the garden looked drier than usual. When I had lived at home, there were days when I would come home from school and walk down the side alley of cracked and uneven concrete to the backyard to see the soil beautifully done with mounds of earth separating each growing patch of squash. It was all so neatly arranged. The soil was always dark and nutritious. Not the case this year. Nonno hadn't been feeling well enough to work his magic.

Having had very little to eat, Nonno immediately went to sit in the chaise rocking chair where he briefly fell asleep. We continued to enjoy the food, the company, and the light breeze that late July day.

"Giuseppina!" A startled expression crossed Nonno's face as he yelled for my aunt. His voice sounded alarmed. Not more than fifteen minutes had passed from the time he had sat down and closed his eyes.

"Was he afraid to die?" I thought, witnessing the horrific look on his face. His voice certainly sounded like he was.

The change in his demeanor from this past Thanksgiving and as recently as May when he came to my daughter Gabriella's third birthday party was astonishing. He seemed tired during the past few months, and had grown fond of a comfortable green upholstered sitting chair that adorned my parent's living room. At family gatherings he spent more time sleeping than usual. At eighty-seven, he seemed to have given up; having lost his spirit to go on living, and often referring to himself as the *vecchiaio*, or old person.

"Ciali," Nonno called to me as he started to rise from the chair. He needed to be helped inside to the bathroom and enlisted my aid. As I supported him from my left, Nonno's arm was around my side. I couldn't escape the thought that I had done this before, only the person I had assisted was different. It was Nonna. As I wandered in thought, my grandfather talked, practically yelled, at me. His thin creviced face was angry. His eyes showed disgust, pleading with me, but knowing it was too late. He talked about the woman he was married to. All I could discern was a comparison between her and the devil. My father came in behind us as we were passing the kitchen sink and he took over for me. By the time they returned from the bathroom, almost twenty minutes had passed.

"De, how did Daddy get those marks on his leg?" my father asked his younger brother Diego, as he settled back in his seat on the hard wooden bench. My father had not seen the large bruises on Nonno's legs before.

"You know how he is. I think he told me he fell, but told me not to say anything to anyone."

I sat quietly on the bench. I felt my neck start to ache from hunching over. There was no back support on my dad's makeshift picnic benches. Besides my aching neck, my shoulders bore the brunt of the tension. I couldn't help but think just how utterly obstinate my grandfather was.

I glanced over my left shoulder only to find Nonno had once again drifted back to sleep. I thought about all my grandfather had been through in his life. My thoughts were suddenly taken over by the realization that despite how warm it was outdoors, Nonno still had on his sweater. As he slept, we talked about him.

"Tell me he looks okay to you," I challenged everyone at the table. On this issue, Lisa agreed with me. He did not look good.

"Tony, you said he was doing fine, he looked good?" Josephine questioned her brother. The reddish frame of her glasses matched the light lipstick she wore, both in stark contrasted to her pale skin.

"Ehh, Josephine what can I tell you?" Tony started in his defense. "To me he looks the same."

"How can you say that, Da?" I jumped in.

Once the words had escaped my lips, I decided to keep quiet and not push the issue because my dad's usually calm demeanor was beginning to show signs of upset. I noticed the increase of gray hairs on his balding head and how my father's face was showing signs of stress and fatigue. His usually happy disposition, like when he first saw his granddaughter in the morning, was missing today.

I got up from the table easing my long legs out from under the wooden structure and over the bench. I picked up some paper plates littered with remnants of hotdogs and buns. A salad leaf dropped onto the stone patio. As I walked to the house, I turned back and whispered, but made sure I spoke loud enough for everyone to hear.

"I give him to the end of the summer."

◆　　◆　　◆

"Hello."

"Heh!" The voice startled me, shaking me from my retrospection and into the present.

"Hello, sorry to disturb you."

It was the respiratory technician, Eduardo, (according to the ID hanging from the left pocket of his coat). He was here to check Nonno's breathing. He spoke to me as he wrote something down on a chart, the pages of which were kept together by a big silver clipboard.

I tried to shake the disoriented feeling of being awaken so quickly. The white-coated technician leaned across the bed railing and placed an oxygen mask over Nonno's face. He explained to me the apparatus would help open my grandfather's bronchial tubes. The machine was no stranger to me since Gabriella and my niece Sabrina had used these nebulizers at home to help each of them deal with their bouts of congestion from bad colds.

Nonno woke up as the thin green elastic band snapped around his head. He mumbled, but without his dentures I couldn't understand him. The expression on his face spoke for him. Nonno was visibly annoyed.

"*Stanco*," he said. His voice sounded dry and parched as he told me he was tired.

"Don't worry, Nonno," I said, trying to be reassuring. I guessed it worked because Nonno went right back to sleep.

The oxygen mask made Nonno look like a dragon. His breathing was labored. I leaned over to pull up the gown, which had fallen from his bony shoulder. His breastbone and ribs jutted out from the thin layer of skin covering his body. He had always been on the thin side since his accident way back when, but today he looked especially skeletal. His cheekbones protruded from his face, while the cavities around his eyes had sunk deeper. His face was a topographical map of hills and valleys, and his bearded stubble was grass and cactus on a dry terrain.

"At least he's not in a lot of pain like Nonna was," I thought to myself as I leaned over the cold, metal bed rail to fix the sheet on the other side. The thought brought me a small sense of relief. Nonna had been in unbelievable pain during her entire illness. I tried hard to remember the little details.

"When did her disease start?" I asked myself. "What was the date?"

I felt guilty for thinking about my grandmother while being here with my grandfather. I had a different relationship with my grandmother and my grandfather knew it. Although I had been so much closer to her than Nonno, I was still sad to be losing the patriarch of the family; my last grandparent. I felt worse off for my father. I knew Dad would miss his father's weekly Saturday morning visits. They had spent countless hours sitting under the canopy of grapevines and the peach tree in the backyard discussing issues. Most of them centering on Martha, the woman Nonno had married and their related problems. There were always problems.

"Thank you," I said to Eduardo as he gathered up the chart and clear plastic tubing. He nodded his head in acknowledgment and left the room.

Reclining back in the beige vinyl visitor chair, a pit had formed in my stomach. I arched my neck to the left and stretched. The deep pull could be felt down to my shoulders and upper arms. Finally, I allowed my head to find repose in the high-back chair. "How many patients had this chair seen?" I wondered. No doubt, this same vinyl clad friend had provided temporary refuge to many a patient's relatives as they kept vigil over their loved one. I knew I was probably one in a long line, and surely not the last. I settled back and closed my eyes and posed the question again.

"When did it start?" I closed my eyes.

4

The Beginning of the End

Those evenings were perhaps the most vivid I had ever experienced. Many years later nothing even came close to the memories of those dark hues of the late autumn sky of 1980. It was one of the things I remembered because I actually had the time to notice the sky and enjoy it. On my walks to Nonna's house, the incredibly beautiful canvas of dark navy and periwinkle blue enveloped me. It was the perfect blend of sunset. Sometimes if I was lucky, the departing daylight would leave mysterious streaks of pink or incandescent red across the azure sky.

The walks after dinner were a nice treat for me, a chance to get out of the house and think about other things going on in my life. Tonight was no different.

After finishing dinner, I had accompanied my dad once again. I went out of the front door and my face was caressed by the cool wind of the early evening. I soaked in the moonlit December sky basking in hues of dark, inviting shades. The scene was as pleasing to the eye as the cool crisp air to my face, although it was a bit sharp as it entered my nose and was sucked down through the back of my mouth.

The glow from the silver street lamps lit the way as trees waved in the light breeze; their last remaining leaves loosening from their sturdy branches. I buried my face in the warmth of my brown turtleneck. My nose picked up the scent of my mother's dinner, which had attached itself to the fibers of my cotton shirt. No sooner had I looked up than I noticed my father was five paces ahead. Keeping up with him was always difficult. He walked fast, long strides for a man of medium height. For every step he took, I took two and then skipped a bit just to keep up.

"So much for trying to enjoy the five-minute walk," I commented under my breath as I adapted to his quick pace. These walks with my dad were to have a direct effect on my stride later on in life. As the years passed, I perfected a quick pace and was as comfortable walking fast even though it seemed my calves might snap from the pressure exerted on them, but it actually hurt more to walk slowly.

The *passegiatas* or walks, with my dad always had a purpose. Usually, as was the case this evening, it was to check in on Nonna and specifically to see whether or not her cough was improving. Over the past week it had been getting deeper and more persistent, causing her to spit up phlegm.

Just three weeks ago, Nonna had joined us on our usual Sunday outing. This was a real treat since she hardly ever accompanied us on our jaunts. No matter where we went, Nonna's house was always the final stopping point and the closure to a usually perfect day. It would not be a Sunday without a stop by my grandmother's for a cup of coffee and pastry, which my aunt Josephine religiously brought home, gratis from her job at the local pastry shop (the same one where I would later work and meet my future wife).

When she joined us on that walk three weeks ago, I noticed her cough.

◆   ◆   ◆

"Where do you want to go today?" Tony asked his children Maria and Charles as they consumed their breakfast. Almost in unison, they answered.

"The airport!" said Charles. "The park!" his sister said equally excited.

The two places Charles loved to visit best were the observation deck at the JFK International Arrivals building to view the jumbos from all different parts of the world take off and land, and a drive up and down Park Avenue.

As his father drove, Charles plastered his face to the small triangular rear window of their baby blue Ventura and picked out the buildings where he someday wanted to live.

Today, however, in a move to exercise parental control, their father decided they would visit Oyster Bay, Long Island to see Teddy Roosevelt's home. That was fine with Charles since they had to pass LaGuardia on both legs of the drive. On the ride east, Charles always made sure he had a window seat on the side facing the airport. On the return, he made sure to sit behind the front passenger side.

Tony called his mother, and asked her if she wanted to join them. Surprisingly, she said, "Yes." She seemed to be all right, but her cough was persistent. To alleviate this, she had some hard candy with her to suck.

After visiting the stately and especially large Victorian mansion that once belonged to Teddy Roosevelt, Nonna and her grandson took a seat on one of the many benches that lined the long, winding, tree-lined path leading to the house. Nonna placed her black pocketbook, or borsa, on her lap. She opened the thick metal gold clasp located at the top, reached in with her aging fingers—all but bare save for a plain gold band on her wedding finger—and pulled out her signature candy: Perugina's Glacia mints.

They were a rectangular, opaque hard mint candy about an inch-long wrapped in green and clear cellophane. The mint was pretty powerful, but oh so good.

As they sat in the coolness of the Sunday afternoon, Charles noticed the cough that shook his grandmother's short frame. Her head with its habitual kerchief, bobbed to and fro with each outburst. As gently as she reached into her pocketbook to pull out the mints, she searched the side pocket of her navy wool coat. Charles wasn't quite sure what she was searching for. The next round of coughing came before she had a chance to pull out the white, eyelet-scalloped handkerchief and put it to her mouth. She dabbed away some phlegm from her lip transferring the yellowish excretion onto the perfect three-inch square cloth.

◆   ◆   ◆

I sat in the kitchen as my dad and grandmother chatted in the darkness of her bedroom. A reflection from the kitchen light bounced off the mirror that hung on the far wall of Nonna's bedroom above the dresser. I sat alone. The smell of *melutsa*, a small fish, which Nonna had prepared for dinner that evening permeated the room. The aroma joined scents of my mother's cooking already embedded in my shirt.

I hated this part of the day. The time right after dinner and being indoors and feeling bloated from what I had just eaten, and then dealing with the constant reminder of my over-indulgence from the smells that lingered. The smells that never seemed to go anywhere but into the clothes and walls. If it weren't for the nightly walks, I would have gone crazy.

My eyes stared through the open bedroom door at my dad and grandmother. They were talking in Italian so I really couldn't understand all that much. It was seven o'clock and Nonna was still dressed in one of her homemade dresses. She came from the bedroom to where I sat keeping the vinyl chair warm. She finished a sentence to my dad with her back toward him. Her dress was short-sleeved, and like the bedroom where she had just emerged, the fabric was a midnight blue. She took a seat next to me. Her wiry black and gray hair full, but completely pushed back. The light played against her face shadowing the angles and crevices.

Her back was to the wall and she casually laid her hands on her thighs. Her dark dress and dark features provided a sharp contrast to the kitchen's plain beige walls. The kitchen door exiting to the backyard was to her left.

"I go to the hospitale," she said. "Justta to check myya cough. You comma and visit me?" Her hand patted my left knee. She coughed, her legs straight out in front of her. Her square black shoes shiny.

"Of course," I told her, reacting as if there was nothing to be alarmed about.

As promised, my dad and I visited her in the hospital on January 21, 1980. It was the same day she was admitted and a biopsy taken.

We walked into the nondescript double-bed room, passed the empty bed, and over to Nonna occupying the bed closest to the window. We found her staring at the darkness through the glass. The view was nothing more than the brick wall of the next wing a few feet away. The white, crisp sheets were pulled up around her chest. The only visible parts of her body were her head and arms.

Nonna looked good. I shoved the cord to the nurse's buzzer out of the way and bent over the metal railing.

"Hi, Nonna." I felt the warm touch of her cheek against mine as I squinted in the brightness of the overhead lighting jumping off the white walls and sheets. As Dad spoke to her in Sicilian, I studied her face—an outside observer to their conversation. Seeing both of them there, I realized how much my dad and grandmother were alike in persona and in the way they spoke.

The only word I was able to make from the entire conversation was 'biopsy.' I knew what that meant. She was pointing to her chest. Her fingers told the story of where the doctors had made a cut to take out the tissue to be tested.

After that brief hospital stay, she seemed fine. There was no further mention of her ailment and I took this as a one time isolated incident. Little did I know that I would soon become all too familiar with these halls.

Little by little over the course of the next few months, I came to find out that my grandmother's surgery five years earlier was not for removal of her gallbladder, but a hysterectomy. Being only eight at the time, I wouldn't have known the significance of this surgery, but now everything was slowly piecing together.

With the exception of Nonna's biopsy, the remainder of 1980 was uneventful. The family was very excited about my aunt Josephine's wedding in August. It was an event Nonna looked forward to, and one that took her mind off her illness.

5

1980

Nineteen eighty was not a good year for either Nonna or me. While she was in the fight of her life *for* her life, I was combating my own personal and painful conflict. Although not terminal, it might as well have been. Everything in my life had started to come undone. Along with my concerns about Nonna came the day-to-day reality and struggle just to make it in my freshman year of school.

Josephine's wedding day was humid and muggy, typical for late August. Worse, the air conditioner in the catering hall was not functioning properly. With all the dancing and reveling, I was sweated out by the end of the evening. Within a week my lungs had filled up with water and I was diagnosed with bronchitis. I had never felt such pressure to breathe before.

Missing those first critical weeks of school definitely set me back, and made it so much more difficult for me to fit in and get to know people. A cripplingly shy teenager, making friends was already a huge challenge for me. In the weeks I missed classes, friendships had already formed and I was the odd man out.

High school was a daily struggle. I missed most of my freshman year because I thought people were talking and making fun of me. I was the kid always picked last for a team and often sat alone in the bleachers. This was indicative of my life up to that point. Socially, my life was spent on the bench watching other kids play; the more popular ones, those with lots of friends. While I blamed my predicament on not being in school from day one, I knew it went deeper than that.

I never felt like I fit in anywhere. My introverted personality coupled with my low self-esteem made it difficult for me to strike up conversations, not just in school, but with kids on my block. All too often my peers made their minds up about me even before they had a chance to really know me. In grammar school I was the subject of taunts. Nevertheless, when arriving at school each morning I tried to fit in with the other boys talking about the latest hockey game, sports or whatever.

◆   ◆   ◆

"What did you think of the game?" Kevin asked Auggie. The boys were leaning against the wall of the light brick building. Charles had walked up and stood nearby trying to jump into bits and pieces of the conversation.

"Pretty good," Charles nervously answered Kevin's question.

Charles was smart and knew enough to buy the morning newspaper or catch the sports highlights on the radio to obtain game results or a big play or two before he left for school. He hated that time right before school started where everyone stood idly chatting. The cliques huddled in circles refusing to let anyone in on their conversations. For Charles, finding a group who would allow entry was difficult, and this was only grammar school. So he generally tried to latch on and appear he was with a group by hanging about in the background.

The two boys looked at Charles condescendingly. Their white shirts and standard uniform of gray pants and tie hid their demonic qualities.

"Name two of the Rangers," Auggie challenged Charles.

Charles' mind raced. He knew. He had to know two names. But before he could respond, he was cut down.

"Just as I figured," his classmate chided him.

◆   ◆   ◆

I shook my head as I recalled these memories of my not so pleasant childhood. I hated being exposed to the whims of others and hated myself for not fitting in. I was a social misfit. My paranoia caused me to miss close to three months of school my freshman year. More disconcerting, I had sunk to depths so low, I was doing things I myself could not believe.

Every morning I woke up panic-stricken and sick to my stomach at the thought of going to school. It had become so problematic that my dad had resorted to driving me and dropping me off at the high school gate. Dad would stay at the entrance to ensure I entered the building. The sound of the hard metal doors as I opened them made me want to vomit. On the days where it just wasn't possible for Dad to drop me off, he enlisted my grandfather's assistance.

◆   ◆   ◆

Nonno and Charles walked the length of Ditmars Boulevard. While other kids were walking in groups and laughing and doing things kids did with friends, Charles walked with his head down for fear and embarrassment that someone would see him walking with his grandfather. As they made a right turn and headed up the gently sloping hill of Twenty-seventh Street, Charles wanted so much not to be there. But where else could he go?

"Okay, Nonno, thank you." Charles turned to his grandfather and shook his hand.

"Okay, va a scuola," Nonno said, telling Charles to go to school.

"You don't have to wait for me to go in," Charles said, hoping his grandfather would turn around and head back down that hill. Instead, much to Charles' fear, Nonno waited. His father had no doubt told him to wait until Charles went into the building.

"You can go." Charles insisted, motioning with his hand for Nonno to go down the block. Charles turned and headed down the gravel walkway to the school doors. There were a few people running on the track of the large open area beyond the left wing of the building. As Charles glanced back over his left shoulder he saw Nonno still standing against the ten-foot gray metal gate. Nonno's pants matched the gate nicely. He waved to Charles.

Managing a faint wave in return, Charles disappeared inside the building, but didn't go far.

He leaned against the cold tiled walls for thirty seconds, and then peered out from the darkened windows of the door. He could see Nonno's baby blue shirt through the mesh of fence thirty yards away as the old man headed down the hill.

Now was his chance!

Charles bolted through the doors and back up the drive, past the fence and then down the hill. He could see Nonno a block ahead of him. Charles turned right on Thirty-first Street and headed for the train, while Nonno took a different route straight up Ditmars.

Charles found a quarter in his pocket and called the school from the train station.

"Hello, this is Mrs. Alaimo," he feigned his mother's voice. "My son Charles will not be attending school today, he's sick."

"Okay Charles, we'll mark you absent," a voice on the other end of the phone told him.

He was aghast! Christ, they recognized him. When he slammed down the receiver he knew he was in for it. But he would have plenty of time to think about his action during the day. That feeling of emptiness grew as Charles began his ascent up the stairs to catch the train into Manhattan—his sanctuary.

On the days he skipped school, going home was not an option. Wandering the streets for seven hours didn't really appeal to him either. So the question was where to go? Somehow, he ended up at a place that seemed a natural choice—St. Patrick's Cathedral. And so with his backpack, a few dollars and a token, he made the church his hideout; a hideout from more than just his family, but from the realities he could not face.

Each time he arrived at the large Gothic cathedral, he dipped his hand in the marble holy water font and made the sign of the cross before going to the St. Anthony shrine just past the small gift shop that sold saint cards and statues, most of which he had already collected. He searched for a small white candle in the boxes underneath the iron-trellised scaffolding that held the burning votives; each one representing a prayer or a wish.

He placed a new candle in one of the holders, grabbed a long wooden stick and touched one end to the flame of a burning candle until the narrow stick was alight. All the while the massive organ in the cathedral played a solemn harmony. He made the sign of the cross again and kissed his forefinger as was customary. Charles' prayers always consisted of the same intercession, to give him the strength and courage to face his fears. It had been four months and he was still waiting for some sign.

Each morning, besides the nervousness of his stomach, was the ritual of his prayers. Before leaving for school Charles would go into his room and close the door. From his middle dresser drawer he would pull out a book overflowing with cards and spread them across his neatly made bed. Before him lay a multitude of saint prayer cards. There were so many choices. Would it make more sense to pray to Saint Jude, saint of the impossible or to Saint Anthony? Charles would kneel at the foot of his bed and look up at the picture of the Sacred Heart on the wall five feet above his headboard. He would pray to as many saints as possible in the five minutes he had before leaving for school.

Today, Charles took 'his' seat in the church. He always sat in the same pew, ninth row back on the right side of the main aisle behind the huge ribbed marble column the width of three men. On an ordinary day he sat through no less than three Masses and received communion only once.

The hours passed slowly so it gave him plenty of time to think. He often wondered what others thought of him just sitting there with his backpack next to him. He was always afraid of the truancy officers, but had never seen them. He figured he was no doubt at the top of their list. But Charles was comfortable they would never find him here among the intricately patterned stained-glass windows depicting glorious scenes of Jesus and Mary.

Then there were the other stain-glassed scenes like the one of Saint Rita dressed in her black robe and habit, her head capped with a crown of thorns. Her eyes conveyed abandonment. It was in these scenes he found solace and comfort. His life was much like those in the depictions—full of suffering. But why? He had read in one of his many religious books that to suffer was to become Christ-like, to become closer to God. Sometimes this knowledge made all the challenges and difficulty he faced seem plausible.

But he was sick of not having a normal childhood. He was tired of always being fearful.

"Two o'clock," he said to himself looking at his watch. Grabbing his blue canvas backpack, he threw it over his left shoulder and left Saint Patrick's. His shoes squeaked as he walked along Fifth Avenue.

Charles left the church the same time every day allowing him enough time to walk up Fifth Avenue and catch the train. He would be home by three, perfect timing since school let out at two forty-five.

He had gotten off the train at Ditmars one day and while going down the stairs he decided not to go straight home, but to stop at his grandmother's house.

She answered the door.

"Ehh Ciali!" she kissed him. Her mocha brown dress was creaseless. "Howsa schoola?"(How's school?) She patted his right arm and they walked into the kitchen. "Sitta down," she instructed him. "Che voi a bevere?" (What would you like to drink?) She headed for the white refrigerator. Charles sat down on the low back, brown Formica chair. He felt uneasy.

"Nothing Nonna, just water."

She walked over and handed him a small cup of water, the glass rim encircled with yellow and red flowers. She took a seat across from her grandson in the corner by the window. The lace curtains touched her bare arms softly.

"So, schoola good?"

"Yeah," he had to think of something that sounded like he actually did go to school. "We're going on a trip tomorrow…to the museum."

"Yeah?" Her eyebrows shot up. She found the news interesting. "Aspetta." She instructed him to wait.

She went into her bedroom, and to the right center drawer of the dresser pulled out a blue purse. He was feeling a sudden sense of guilt. Now he had lied to his grandmother.

"You buyya sometinga tomorrow," she said, as she handed him a bill.

From the corner of his right eye he detected movement beyond the hallway. Some-one was at the front door. It was his dad.

Charles heard the buzzer and walked down the corridor to answer the door. On his way he checked out the bill in his hand. "Wow!" he thought. "Five dollars."

Charles' father was upset.

"Where were you today?" his father yelled, his voice rising incrementally with each word as he closed the storm door behind him.

Charles turned around and walked quickly back to the kitchen. He didn't know how to respond to his father's question. His father was so angry and knew if Nonna had not been there he would have surely gotten a quick, hard kick to his ass.

Charles sat down across from Nonna. His father continued yelling, his voice echo-ing in the open rooms.

"Mommy got a call from the school again and said you didn't show up." He raised his arms out in front of him. "They said you phoned in sick. What's going on, Char-lie?"

"Okay, okay calmati." Nonna told her son to calm down.

At this point Charles was more embarrassed than fearful, not because of his father's bellowing, but because he was caught in a lie to Nonna. Never had he done anything like this before. Shameful, he disappeared into the basement as his father told his mother in their native language that Charles was a no good for nothing.

Two minutes later Charles heard footsteps. Nonna was coming down the stairs.

He saw her legs first, and then noticed her black shoes land on each step. Her foot-steps were slightly muffled because of the brown rubber stair pads on the thirteen wooden steps. She emerged into view and saw her grandson sitting in a recliner. Her steps were noticeably harsher on the hard tiled floor as she approached him.

"Whya you lie a to me?"

"I'm sorry," Charles said, extending his hand with the five-dollar bill she had just given him ten minutes before.

"No, you keepa," she said, pushing his hand back toward him. "Butta you no lie a no more, okay?"

"Okay," he said without looking up.

He stood and she put her arm around him. As they hugged, he looked straight over her right shoulder. On the wall underneath the staircase hung a simple picture of Our Lady of Sorrows. Her dark blue robe was clasped about her neck. Her downcast eyes conveyed disappointment and desolation.

Unfortunately, Charles had missed so much school that year the only way they would take him back was if he scheduled an appointment and be assessed by the school psychologist. They found nothing seriously wrong with him after he had spilled his *guts. He was put on Valium and much to his amazement he managed to finish out the year.*

◆   ◆   ◆

During this time in my life, the one thing I looked forward to more than anything else was the weekends. On Saturdays I could finally relax and not be made fun of at school. The stresses of daily life were given a respite for a brief forty-eight hours.

I wanted to do as much as possible to make the weekends last. I always made sure of a full day on Saturday. Those days often started pretty early; helping my father do some task around the house, whether it was breaking down a wall here, digging out a basement there. When Saturday night rolled around and I thought about Sunday, my stomach would twinge.

I usually spent Saturday night sleeping over at Nonna's. I had found a refuge in her house; solace for all the pain I was feeling. Being there on the weekends was the best medicine. However, Sunday inevitably rolled around and once again, thoughts of the next day. The roller coaster feeling started in the pit of my stomach. I wanted Sundays to last forever.

They never did.

6

A New and Strange Word

With the passing of 1980, one of the worse years of my life, I was finally coming to grips with my problems, although my issues and concerns constantly consumed my thoughts. I was tired of always being fearful, of the talking behind my back, of not fitting in. It was a great feat for me to even feign I was having a good time at weekend gatherings or at a party in the company of my own family, for my thoughts followed me everywhere making me a prisoner of depression and anxiety.

I did not know what it meant to be relaxed in a setting. As basic as it sounds that was all I wanted; to feel what it was like to be carefree and worry free. Despite all I was dealing with personally, I did not fail to notice that something was not quite right with the most important person in my life. It was in January, 1981 while accompanying Nonna home that I first noticed her walk was off.

Earlier that month my younger sibling, Mark had broken his leg during a roller skating outing with his class. With everyone gone and working, my grandmother was the one who came over each and every day to supervise my eleven-year-old brother.

"You okay, Nonna?" I asked as we walked. My left arm was entwined with her right, her gray coat warm against my bare hand.

"Justta a little pain." She seemed pensive, her eyes looked straight ahead.

Her kerchief pulled her hair tight beneath the floral and blue wrap. Her step wasn't sure and she limped slightly. Not more than a few days after that walk I heard she was going back to the doctor to have the pain checked out. My worse fears were confirmed when that visit revealed her cancer was back. This time in her bones, and already showing signs of infiltration through her leg.

At thirteen, there was a new word in my vocabulary.

Terminal.

7

Blissful Ignorance

It was appropriate that I found out my grandmother was dying in such a matter-of-fact sort of way. Much like Nonna's life, which was ordinary, so too was the news that her time would soon be coming to an end. It came on a summer day during one of her many doctor visits.

As was the standard, Aunt Olivia was coming to pick up Nonna and me as she had done on so many days this summer. I arrived early to make sure that if Nonna needed help, which she always did, that I was there.

The wait was excruciating. In the short span of time between getting ready and being picked up, it was awkward since we couldn't really start anything that might take too much time. There was not much to do outside of sitting in the kitchen or waiting by the door, as was the case today, and peering through the glass storm door.

I stood next to my grandmother and noticed she was unusually quiet. She was dressed in a mocha brown sleeveless dress with a hem that ended just below her knees. The powder she had sprinkled on her body just a few hours before was evident right below her armpits where it had smudged lightly into the brown material. Her black hair, showing just a trace of gray, was nicely brushed. Her eyes were distant. Her fingers gently patted the silver tubing of her walker while her head swung back and forth as she looked up and down the block.

Clara and Agnes, the neighbors two doors down, walked past as they went to the house they shared. Nonna waved at them through the glass door. Although they were sisters, they couldn't have been more different. Clara was short and hunched. Her hair was a bunch of wild gray, like unkempt rosebushes that had grown strong from years of neglect and lack of pruning. When my siblings and I played in the common alleyway in back of Nonna's house, Clara would always watch us and laugh.

Agnes, on the other hand, was tall and thin, the sensible one. She kept her hair smartly short and close to her face. She reminded me of a librarian or the typical school marm. From Nonna's stoop in the backyard, they could often be seen lunching and talking. For me there was always comfort in seeing them eating together or enjoying a cup of coffee and taking in each other's company. They were nice neighbors.

Nonna's head followed them. I watched her eyes as she watched them walk by. The sadness was evident in her gaze. I looked down toward my sneakers feeling incredibly helpless. If I could have had one wish right then it would have been to make her walk, to make this horrible disease that was robbing her of her most basic freedoms to go away.

"Clara," she said softly. Her left hand reached up and her creased fingers extended across the window. Her plain gold wedding band shown brightly in the sun as her fingertips gently touched the glass when the two old sisters passed. Of course they couldn't hear her.

The block was slowly changing. Old familiar neighbors being replaced with new people who didn't want to be bothered with knowing who lived next door. The small tightknit block was unraveling like a ball of Nonna's yarn she kept in her sewing kit.

Of all her current and former neighbors, I knew Nonna missed Senora Nanetta the most. She and her husband Mr. Charlie had returned to Sicily not more than six months ago. They had been next-door neighbors for as long as I could remember, and both were the nicest people you'd ever want living next to you.

Nanetta's smile was genuine, showing lots of teeth and a space in her upper right quadrant. Mr. Charlie, as he was called, had owned a small barbershop on Twenty-third Avenue where I had frequented as a young child. He was a small man with spectacles and a balding head that reminded me of Gepetto. Whatever hair he had left encircled the circumference of his head from ear to ear. They lived with their daughter, son-in-law and two grandchildren.

Nanetta had dark features. Her hair was black with a fair amount of gray mixed in. Her powerful voice carried when she spoke, and was just as loud as the sleeveless black and red flowered sundresses she often wore. If my family and I were visiting Nonna and chatting under the grapevines of the small concrete patio, we always knew when Nanetta was on her way up the basement stairs to the backyard by the heavy thumping of her black wedged slip-ons.

As I leaned up against the cool marble of the hallway entry wall, I laughed to myself when I remembered Senora Nanetta and a dish of fried rice she had brought over for us to try one Saturday. It was the first fried rice I had ever eaten. Since my dad did not believe in eating out and always insisted on home cooked meals, I did not know what it meant to eat in a restaurant. My experience with cuisine, outside of my mother or grandmother's cooking, was limited to say the least.

I had certainly never eaten Chinese food before, but to me that experience was an eye-opener. It would be years before I realized that authentic fried rice did not contain chopped hot dogs. Still, the rice that Saturday was exotic and very tasty and I liked it.

Nonna often had to give Senora Nanetta her insulin shots, which explained why the two of them often disappeared into Nonna's bedroom while I was visiting.

It was great having them live next door. We regularly sat in my grandparent's yard chatting under the clear blue skies of spring or summer. Nanetta and her clan often joined in on the conversation through the chainlink gate that separated us.

The small patch of neatly kept concrete was perfect to accommodate four lounge chairs. The green garden hose was coiled up close to the house and to the right of the large basement window. Having coffee and cake out there with company was always special. The departure of our favorite neighbors was depressing for Nonna and for me as well. Things were changing and I sensed deep in my heart that these changes were not for the better.

I could see Aunt Olivia's burgundy sedan coming down the block. Her shiny car with bright silver rims sparkled as she pulled up alongside the parked cars in front of the house. She honked the horn. I had already opened the storm door and had it resting on my backside as I eased Nonna down the first step to the large top landing. The warm summer breeze greeted us as we left the house.

Although I was young and naive in many ways, I could feel the sense of burden on my aunt at having to constantly drive the two of us to the myriad of scheduled appointments.

"Josephine goes to work. She should be taking your grandmother to the doctors," she once told me.

At the time I wasn't sure what she expected me to say. I certainly did not want to create waves, so kept my thoughts and comments to myself.

Today Nonna had a cobalt treatment that took us to a doctor's office way up on Queens Boulevard right past Alexander's department store. I had no idea what the hell cobalt treatments were. All I knew is that doctors drew on her legs with a heavy black marker. There was a square here and there, and long rectangles on her right leg. It reminded me of one of those butcher posters showing the cow dissected by thick, black lines depicting the choicest cuts.

Much later I learned that during these different visits, Nonna was given radiation in a specific area of her leg, which explained the markings.

Before she started down the flight of sixteen steps leading from her front door to the bottom landing, I grabbed the walker and ran down the steps to where my aunt was waiting. When I ran back up, Nonna was already holding onto the iron railing with her right hand. She placed her left arm gently around my shoulders. I hunched over just a bit since I was a good foot taller than she, and placed my right arm around her waist and off we went.

We took each step carefully. Nonna couldn't leave one foot on the step while the other was on its way down. Instead, when her right foot made its way to the step below, it would have to wait for her left one to join it. Once her black-heeled feet were together the process was repeated. Upon reaching the bottom, I allowed Nonna to walk the distance from the front gate to Aunt Olivia's car. She liked not having to use the walker, even if only for a few minutes.

I would have to repeat this process when we arrived at the doctor's office. It was tiring but I had it down pat. I did not complain. I did it for Nonna. Her pain and suffering were enough to put it all in perspective. For me it was the least I could do to feel I was helping her in some way.

Upon reaching the doctor's office, we entered the front door of the three-family house and waited our turn in the small, rather cramped waiting lounge. A few minutes had passed when Nonna's neighbor, Mrs. LaRosa, emerged from the staircase leading up from the treatment center in the basement. I thought it utterly ridiculous the patients had to go down, and worse yet, climb back up this long and steep flight of stairs to the examination rooms.

Nonna knew Mrs. LaRosa had cancer, so I wondered if she had made the connection. If she did, she kept it to herself when they exchanged pleasantries.

When Nonna went downstairs for her treatment, Aunt Olivia engaged me in conversation.

"You know Charlie, they givva your grandma maybe two or three monthsa atta most," she said in her heavy Sicilian accent.

I just looked at her. This was the first time anyone had communicated this news to me. I would have rather heard this from someone else other than my aunt who seemed to deliver it in quite a harsh and insensitive manner considering I was only fifteen-years-old then. Reality hit me hard in the face that day.

"But was I really that surprised?" I questioned myself. "Was I really that naive to think that Nonna was going to come out okay from all this?"

I blamed myself for being so out of it. I should have known her cancer was more serious than I had been told. Perhaps for this very reason I did not give much thought to her demise. I never saw her death as an option.

I returned home early from my grandmother's that day. I cried all the way home. My mom had told my father when he got home from work that I was very upset.

"Just pray to God," Dad told me. "But don't cry."

"How utterly stupid," I said under my breath after my father had left my room. My face buried in my pillow, I chose to ignore him. I could feel my eyes were swollen and my nose was running all over my yellow pillowcase. I was tired and my faced was soaked, but I think I was more upset at my father for seeming to blow all this off as if Nonna's illness was nothing to be greatly concerned about. It was just like my father to say something like that. His answer to everything was to pray to God. To me, this was my father's way of burying his head in the sand and dealing with the inevitable. My father was exactly like his father. They both avoided and ignored anything that was too tough to deal with. This time, however, I was not convinced that praying to God was the answer. Nonna had done plenty of that herself and to no avail. I was annoyed at my father for not allowing me to grieve or even participate in a discussion of Nonna's fate.

Dad was like this with everyone. There were way more examples I could think of. One was Saturday, September 5, two days before Nonna was admitted to the hospital. This was to be her last visit.

◆   ◆   ◆

All the siblings were present. This fifth day of September was cooler; a sign that hopefully the hot weather was breaking.

Josephine, Diego and Tony, were in the bedroom. This had not been a good day for Nonna. She was in a lot of pain and crying incessantly.

Humidity hung in the air. From Charles' vantage point in the kitchen it was more uncomfortable inside the house than outside. With no air conditioning, the humidity only made Nonna feel worse.

"Ai Ai." She bit her lip and grimaced hard as she tried to prop herself higher on the pillow.

Her children had tried moving her to make her more comfortable in bed. Besides the cancer, her bedsores had grown worse too. Charles continued to stand in the kitchen, his back propped up against the sink. He could feel the Formica lip of the counter digging into the small of his back. Through the back screen door he could see

Mark and Maria playing on the pathway in the yard, oblivious—probably for the better—to what was happening inside.

Nonna began crying even more, her arms shook in the sleeveless white nightgown. She hurt from the cancer and from the horrendous bedsores that had eaten away at her back. Josephine was to the left of the bed in full view from the doorway. She leaned over and held onto Nonna's arm trying to pull her closer to that side of the bed. Nonna grimaced, her face creviced with lines, and her upper teeth bit into her bottom lip. Her hair was unwashed and unmade. Coupled with the heat and her sweat, her hair was greasy. Strands of hair pointed upward away from her face.

Before Charles realized what was happening, Josephine rushed by him running out of the bedroom and down to the basement. She was sobbing hysterically. No more than ten seconds later Tony followed, composed as always. Charles shifted several feet to his left, closer to the basement doorway to better listen.

"Josephine, you can't cry in front of Mommy," Tony reprimanded his younger sister as if she had done something terribly wrong.

"How utterly lame," Charles thought as he shook his head. "What good was it not to cry?"

Josephine and Tony walked back up from the basement five minutes later. Josephine's eyes were incredibly red and swollen behind her gold-framed lenses.

◆   ◆   ◆

Over the years, Dad dealt with grief in much the same way. For example, when my mom was diagnosed with breast cancer, not once did he ever truly discuss the ramifications with me and my siblings. The only discussion we had was a chat at the dining room table where he told us everything was going to be all right, and then he looked to me for validation.

Both my parents were funny that way. They weren't the type to show a lot of emotion. By emotion I mean talking about pain, sharing grief, showing me it was okay to cry. For my mom, I figured this was her safety mechanism. Her mother had a stroke when she was only thirteen and her father 'brainwashed' her, for lack of a better word, into thinking she was going to hell for "not having Christ in her life."

I had only met the man, a born-again Christian and whom I always referred to as 'my mother's father,' a handful of times. The only time I was able to recall was a dinner at my parent's house. My only memory was of him going on and on about Jesus. He did call a lot though. I hated answering the phone when he was on the other end. I hated being told by a man who had remarried and never visited his family that we were all going to hell.

I remembered coming across a black and white photo taken when my mom was young. She was conspicuously the only girl in a room full of fat old men, supposedly at a Bible discussion given by her father in their house. When I saw things like this I could see why my mother was the way she was. I was glad he didn't call often and even happier I had maintained my distance from him.

◆   ◆   ◆

There was now a new sense of isolation. There was not one person I could turn to and discuss what was happening with Nonna. What did the future look like? With nobody willing to engage in any real conversation as to my grandmother's fate, it was up to me to come to terms with her illness in my own way.

Once I knew the severity of her illness, I played a game with myself. On my daily trips to visit her, I envisioned she was not there. On one visit as she walked down the hallway from the kitchen, her back toward me, I sat in the low-backed dining room chair and watched her intently. I tried to emblazon her navy dress, her black shoes, even the sounds of them lifting ever so gently off the floor, and then hitting the beige and brown blocked linoleum as they came down, all to memory. I imagined a house with no sound. No block heels slipping across the floor. No light moans or the tapping of the rubber walker feet against the floor.

I would close my eyes and try to picture her in my head, as if in an instant photo. But I had one big problem. How would I keep the sound of her voice with me after she was gone? I hadn't yet quite figured that out.

With each visit the diversion continued with the goal of capturing her movements, her expressions, and her touch. I was creating a mental scrapbook. Hopefully, I would be able to go back to it when she was gone and open those pages in my mind.

I tried to commit everything to memory. The hug, the kiss hello I received when she welcomed me every day. The feel of her skin when I patted her shoulder. Each and every aspect of her ordinary, daily life was vital to me in keeping her memory alive.

8

A Grandson's Mission

Today, Wednesday, June 17, 1981 was another doctor visit. They were all becoming a blur. Nonna was going to her oncologist. Before I knew it, we were pulling up in front of the aqua blue doorway of the two-story home where the doctor's office occupied the first floor.

The minutes flew by while we sat in the rather spacious waiting room. My grandmother was preoccupied with waiting to be called. She didn't catch my gaze as I studied her face. She was busy looking around at the other patients and probably wondering why they were here.

She wore the light brown dress she had made herself. She sat upright in the chair. The muscles and fat on her arms sagged as she extended them over the top of her walker. Her hair was nicely done around her face, and with the exception of a few gray areas, the majority was still original black. Things could have been much worse for her. I knew this all too well. She could have lost all her hair from the chemo or lost an incredible amount of weight and be like one of those human skeletons barely surviving. Surely the saints who Nonna prayed to each day had a hand in ensuring that she suffered from none of these cruel symptoms of 'getting better.'

Her name was finally called. Aunt Olivia assisted her to the room and stayed with her for the duration of the exam. I waited alone, flipping through pages of magazines. The humidity was so high, the plastic chair stuck to the bare skin on my legs.

I waited for what must have been another forty-five minutes. Finally, my aunt returned to the waiting area. That was my signal to get up from the uncomfortable brown plastic chair, now warm thanks to my rear being on it for nearly two hours.

Knowing my grandmother wouldn't be far behind my aunt, I turned into the dark hallway leading to the examination rooms just as Nonna was exiting. Her arms were bent at the elbow, her fingers firmly grasping the walker. She methodically lifted each foot starting from the heel then working toward the toes until the foot was airborne and lifted lightly off the floor. She continued to walk toward me pushing her walker in sync with each step. The hollow silver metal frame clanked each time it hit the floor despite the rubber footings on each of its four legs.

She walked the ten steps toward me and then picked one seat out of the five that lined the wall in the dim hallway and sat down. The pure joy of just sitting was evident on her face. From a small pocket she had conveniently sewn into her dress just below the waistline, she pulled out a small item wrapped in a paper towel. She undid the package to reveal a light brown Bosc pear and gently sunk her teeth into it. The juicy sounds were extremely enticing. I grew thirsty, especially in light of the fact that I hadn't had anything to drink in sometime, and sitting in the waiting room on this warm day was dehydrating. She swallowed her first bite and used the paper towel to dab the little bit of liquid that dripped from her chin.

"Ciali," she reached out and patted my right forearm. Her fingers were cold from the pear she held in her hand.

"Yeah, Nonna?"

She motioned me closer with her head. Her eyes glanced to where my aunt stood talking with the doctor.

"Go and listen, *a che dice il dottore.* (to what the doctor is saying)" A smirk crossed her face, her eyes pleaded with a note of mischievousness.

Being the good grandson that I was, I obliged and went back into the bright waiting room. Emerging from the darkness of the hallway, the iridescent light hurt my eyes. The lights made up for what was missing from the weather that day. Besides being muggy, it was a gray day with no sunlight. I thought of how much it reminded me of the typical summer day right before thunderous storms and rains, which according to the forecast were actually going to develop later on that day.

I tried to overhear what they were saying while keeping an eye on Nonna. Although her taste buds had long lost their function, I could clearly tell she was enjoying that pear. She held onto it as if it were her salvation. She glanced to where I stood by the front desk. Her eyes told me she appreciated me gathering information on her behalf.

"Did she think someone was trying to keep information from her?" I thought to myself.

I became aware of the sweat dripping from my underarms onto my beige tank top.

"Okay, so more treatments," I heard Aunt Olivia speak through the din of the ringing phones and the receptionist saying, "Hello, doctor's office."

I returned without any earth shattering news.

"Che? What?" Nonna asked.

"Nothing, *niente* Nonna," I said, shrugging my shoulders as I jammed my hands deeper into the pockets of my navy blue canvas shorts. "They are just talking about your next appointment." I looked away.

"Oh, okay," she said.

She seemed pleased and took another bite of her tasteless pear.

9

Providenza

There was nothing more depressing for me to think about than my grandmother being alone. I knew the feeling of being alone, and wished I had someone much like myself to worry about me. I guess for the most part, Nonna was that person for me, as I was to her. She cared about me and let me know it. I liked it when she asked me how my day went at school. I liked the way she patted the seat of a chair indicating for me to come sit next to her. Outside of Nonna, there wasn't much in the way of people who really showed any interest in me. My role of the provider, the helper, and the confidante disguised much of my own pain.

Like much of that summer, my activities were already planned for me. They almost always went something like: wake up, take a bath, eat breakfast, and go to Nonna's. Monotony had set in, but it was okay with me. Besides, I had little else to do that summer. My social life, or lack of it, was the end result of my introversion. It wasn't just awkward silence at having to start up a conversation or to introduce myself. My sense of self-worth was even more diminished in the one thing I despised most: Gym class. In my opinion, this class had little to do with physical exercise and more to do with exercising superiority.

The same guys were always selected to be team captains of competition games like touch football. They always picked the same guys for their teams, and it was always the same group of kids left remaining—the ones nobody wanted and unfortunately had no choice in the matter. I was always one of them. There was nothing more humiliating than being the last person left sitting on the cold, hard, brightly polished wood floor of the gymnasium and watching the expressions of players who were forced to make me part of their team.

However, there were moments where I proved everyone wrong. One time during a touch football game I intercepted a throw from the other side and without even thinking, as if some miraculous force had come down on me, I fell to one knee on my team's five-yard line. The reaction was overwhelming; first from shock on my part, then from my teammates, and then jubilation. Now mind you, I had little experience to know of such a move, and how I knew to do it I hadn't a clue. But I sure as hell left that gym class feeling good about myself. This was a rarity, however, and I was realistic in knowing that future events like this would be few and far between.

I was left to rely on very few people, and most of those not of the earthly world; namely the same saints my grandmother prayed to each day. I trusted they would never send more my way than I could handle in terms of taunts and difficult situations, but they were letting me down, much the same as they were letting my grandmother down by not allowing her to get better.

Because I was able to assist my grandmother with the most mundane tasks, I felt like I was giving back and making a real difference in her quality of life. More than anything else, I truly believed my presence during the day made all the difference to her. Without me, she had no real company. Besides, it wasn't like I had a hoard of friends calling me away from her.

If it weren't for me taking care of my grandmother my days would have been horrifically boring, and no doubt so to would have Nonna's. So it was probably fortuitous that I had very few friends to hang out with that summer since someone else on a much higher plane had bigger plans for me.

My grandfather was out all the time, either visiting his brother Angelo, or shopping. I came to believe that it was my grandfather's way of avoiding Nonna's illness. By carrying on his daily rituals, he could put off dealing with her illness and therefore refuse to deal with the inevitable. The old adage that 'the apple doesn't fall far from the tree' would apply when it came to his behavior and that of my dad.

Nonno was never a comforter. This was most likely due to his childhood, growing up with a father who showed him little, if any love. I couldn't fault him, but then again Nonna was his wife. Not once did he accompany her to any of the doctor visits, and you could all but forget him doing housecleaning or anything of that nature. His was the traditional European male ideology; housework was meant for women. It was fine by me if he wasn't around, his presence at times only made matters worse.

I happily trudged over to Nonna's this bright July day. The morning sun felt warm against the back of my neck. My legs, at least the part not covered by the long white socks with the band of red just below the knees, benefited from the rays. The sun crept briefly along the left side of my face once I had turned onto Thirty-sixth Street before ultimately disappearing behind the train overpass. The huge concrete arched tunnel supported the rails of Amtrak and long freight trains making their way to points within and beyond the city.

My long hair flopped in my eyes as I inhaled the moist dewy air of morning. For me, the best part of these ordinary days was being greeted at the front door. Nonna, when she was able, would walk with the trusty aid of her metallic companion to let me in. When she opened the wooden, lacquered front door, I peered in through the intricate iron trelliswork of the storm door. I could see past the long entry foyer and hallway, past the kitchen and through the screen door exiting into the backyard.

On this day like so many others, I waited a half-minute or so before ringing the bell, using that time to memorialize the scene through the storm door. The morning light came in through the back door's eastern exposure. My grandmother sat alone with a coffee cup in her hand and looked out into the garden. I wondered what she thought about when she had those quiet moments alone.

After ringing the bell, I had time to capture the way her fingers gripped the gray rubber handles of the cold, shiny walker. The smile on her face knowing I was at the door—a smile that tried desperately to hide grimaces of pain. Her arms shook from the stress of supporting her body. Her loose folds of skin jiggled softly back and forth above her light blue, flowing housedress. It enveloped her lightly, never touching her skin but for the sleeveless part right above her shoulders.

"Ciali." She greeted me with a huge smile and a kiss.

"Good morning," I said, happily returning her greeting as I kissed her right cheek. My arm touched her bare upper arm. She smelled like baby powder.

The disease she was slowly succumbing to showed no visible or outward signs other than robbing her of the ability to walk and the accompanying pain, both physical and mental. Her disposition, her smile, and her laugh all remained intact and unaffected.

There was always plenty of time to chat during the day while doing chores. I placed some magazines I had brought with me on the kitchen windowsill and got quickly to work helping Nonna with the breakfast dishes and tidying up the brown and beige Formica dining table. We often sat at this round table, just talking. The table could easily accommodate four, but it was often pushed into the corner and then only two could sit comfortably.

Nonna slowly walked the short distance from the small dinette to the bedroom. Her slippered feet dragged along the linoleum floor. As each foot moved forward, I could hear the lining of her slippers peeling away from the bottom of her feet (much the same way as if you were to sit on plastic slipcovers in shorts in the middle of summer). I began putting the remainder of the dishes away and turned my head in time to see Nonna drag the ironing board from the huge closet behind the door. I took a step in her direction but stopped. I thought it best if she did something on her own, to feel she was still somewhat independent.

She proceeded to sit at the edge of her high bed. The mattress was extra comfy when you sat on it, but because of Nonna's rather short stature, her feet dangled two inches above the floor. I momentarily stepped away from the sink to run into her bedroom and bend down to plug in the iron for her. It wasn't until I returned to my dishwashing duty that I realized I should have dried my hands first. Luckily, all that remained to be washed were two glasses and a spoon, which I placed in the small basket on the draining board with the spoons and forks.

"You okay, Nonna?" I asked as I peeked into the bedroom.

"Yeah, yeah no worry," she replied.

This time I took the extra step of grabbing a green and white striped dishtowel, and after drying my hands proceeded to wipe the splattered water off the edges of the sink. Afterward, I walked the short distance to the basement stair landing and grabbed the broom. It was wedged against the wall thanks to a wire mesh shopping cart. I grabbed the broom and large metal dustpan and made my way down the hallway then into the kitchen where I checked in with Nonna. She was waiting for the iron to warm-up and was just getting underway with her chores.

I was a great sweeper. I made sure every speck of dust was swept from the floor, and using the broom bristles, even made sure the molding was dust free. My grandmother often directed me from her vantage point in the bedroom. She reminded me to get under the bed, and all the way under the dressers and chairs. I learned never to do a halfway job. I wanted Nonna to approve of everything I did.

She always did.

◆   ◆   ◆

There was a Saturday that summer of 1981, when Charles' sister Maria came to help him clean their grandparent's house. For Charles it was a nice treat having another able-bodied person to help. Their dad accompanied them, but he was there to help Nonno in the garden.

Charles cleaned Nonna's room and Maria tackled the living room. Maria decided to clean the television first. Before the wooden top could be dusted, she had to remove the antenna and seagull statue. The statue was a souvenir from their parents' honeymoon to Bermuda back in 1964. The foot-long piece depicted a gliding seagull, its gray and white wings fully extended. The base was an aquamarine and sea green ocean wave complete with a whitecap. Maria held the statue with one hand, the other glided over the smooth porcelain finish.

Crash!

Charles' shoulders hunched instinctively as he heard something hard hit the floor in the living room. He gritted his teeth and grimaced hoping it was not anything delicate. The door dividing the living room and Nonna's room was open. He went to the doorway and asked his sister what had happened. Before she could even respond, he saw the broken wing in her hand.

"Shit," he muttered to himself.

Nonna was sitting at the bare kitchen table, while the tablecloth was being washed. The brown Formica edges encircled the large, smooth beige top of the table.

"Che?" Nonna said, asking Charles what happened. She knew something had fallen, but what exactly she hadn't a clue.

Charles went back to the living room.

"Maria," he said. "Just give me the pieces and we'll see if we can put it back together."

Charles thought it best if he carried the broken gull to Nonna for her inspection. He placed it on the table. Nonna grabbed the three-inch tip that sheared off and tried to fit it.

"I'll glue it back, Nonna," Charles said reassuringly as he watched his grandmother fumble with the broken figure. Her eyes became red and watery. He turned his head quickly and saw Maria throw her paper towel in the garbage. Tears flowed from Nonna's eyes, and continued to hold the broken seagull.

"Che Mamma?" Tony said as he came into the kitchen from the backyard and asked his mother what was wrong.

"Dalia!" (Look!) She held up the broken wingtip so her son could see what had happened.

She began to cry lightly, her shoulders jerking up and down with each sob. Charles knew it wasn't the figurine she was crying over, she looked worn and tired today. She hadn't had a chance to bathe and her hair was matted in some places. Nonna was clearly frustrated and aggravated by her illness and by her inability to move, bend, or help with the most menial of chores. Her days were spent in this little kitchen and her bedroom, shuffling from one place to the other. She was owed an opportunity every now and then to let it all out.

"Okay, e niente, no piange," Tony said, telling her not to cry since it was nothing.

She stopped, but her eyes were still swollen. Her head rested on her right hand propped beneath her chin. Her plain gold wedding band seemed tight on her swollen hand.

"*Ciali never breaka nuttinga,*" she said. Uncharacteristically, Nonna let her feelings show as she voiced her displeasure at Maria's cleaning techniques.

After that day, Charles' sister was never again seen even carrying a rag in that house.

◆　　　◆　　　◆

"Ciali, no forgetta undernetha tha dressa," Nonna said. Her finger pointed to the large, mirrored dresser. There were nine draws, three rows of three. Held up by its Queen Anne style legs, the dresser stood five inches off the polished, beige and brown squared linoleum.

Following her instruction, I went over and got down on the floor. My brown shorts did nothing to protect my knees. I pushed the broom underneath getting into every corner. I even went down onto my forearms so I could make certain I had left no particle of dust.

It was only eleven in the morning, but I was already wiped out. After sweeping and doing the dishes, I decided to watch some television. From the living room, Nonna was directly in my line of sight just above the television set and through the open doors of the kitchen. Closed, the doors allowed complete privacy. When the doors were open, as one door usually was during the day to allow sunlight in, they provided openness and a chance to keep an eye on her while I rested on the loveseat in the living room.

Nonna's arm went back and forth across the shirt with the black iron making sure every crease was pressed. There was plenty of time for perfection.

Drrriiinnng!

Nonna's phone, an old black rotary dial type, rang from its perch atop her shiny cherry wood night table. Placing the iron down she reached to grab the black receiver from its cradle, but not before it rang again.

Drrriiinnng!

"Ello," she said in broken Italian dialect.

I thought this would be a good time to break away for a second. I hopped off the loveseat and went down the basement stairs to get the washboard from the bathroom. Nonna would need it later to wash some shirts. The washboard was a remnant from the past; an old wooden frame surrounded the thick glass and metal of the scrubber panel. I fetched the rectangular board and decided to climb up the short staircase from the basement to the backyard. I placed the board by the door of the kitchen. Nonna often washed clothes at the backyard stoop.

That stoop was the place where we often gathered informally to chat. The two-foot long wall lining the three steps provided some additional seating when no chairs were available.

Nonna was still on the phone when I entered the kitchen from the yard. I was a bit out of breath. I wondered who was on the phone as I made my way back into the living room. I took in a deep breath of the cool air and wished I could sit outside, but I did not want to be segregated from Nonna in case she needed me.

Whoever was on the other end of the line made her laugh a lot. I was happy about this. These bits of conversation got her through the day and she looked forward to the phone calls she received. In some of the conversations her laughter gave way to somber tones. On some occasions, as was the case with this conversation, tears followed. Sitting there on the edge of the bed, her elbow on the ironing board, the sun behind her, and her failing legs dangling below, I could well understand the tears.

On a day like this, the sun still rising and the sky a beautiful shade of cobalt blue, she would have been walking to Key Food carrying her large plastic shopping bag, the one with the big blue flowers and blue handles to match. Or she would perhaps be taking a walk to church after morning Mass to avoid the crowds and say a prayer and light a candle or two. (I found out much later that my grandmother suffered from anxiety when around crowds, and had a bit of claustrophobia much like what I suffered.) But today found her confined to the four rooms she called home. Her scenery changed only when visitors came and went.

One of Nonna's more colorful guests was Angelina Bellavia. I was six when I first met Angelina. With a name like that I expected a woman with a heavy Italian accent. Quite to my amazement she spoke perfect English. Standing at a mere five feet two inches, she was shorter than my grandmother. Her hair, completely and utterly silver, was always pulled back in a perfect bun. With her coiffed gray hair against the navy backdrop of her dress and wool overcoat, there was something uniquely distinguished about her.

Like Nonna, her feet were always adorned with highly polished, low-heeled black shoes. Even with the one-inch heels, Angelina was a good inch shorter than Nonna.

A special treat during these rare visits was Nonna's coffee that she prepared in the old silver percolator. The smell of the rich blend wafted through the house as we gathered to hear stories and enjoy biscotti. Angelina always brought the biscotti.

Like gentle breezes that punctuated the air of those stifling summer days for only a few precious seconds, Angelina's visits always ended too soon. There was nothing more special and more inviting for Nonna and me than these unexpected visits. There was a sense of depression when it was time for Angelina to head back home to Manhattan. The refreshing respite had come and gone, distracting us for a few priceless hours.

◆   ◆   ◆

With so many household chores to fill the day the hours seemed to fly by. I was always busy, but in a good way. Before I knew it, it was time for lunch and I took the liberty of preparing mortadella sandwiches. I carefully pulled the thin slices of meat from the white deli wrapper and placed them on the hand-torn pieces of Italian bread. At times I even spread a dollop of peanut butter across the speckled Italian cold cut.

"Nonna, do you want soda or water?" I asked my grandmother from the kitchen.

"Aqua," she replied, stating she wanted water.

I poured myself a glass of 7-Up, the only soda she kept in her refrigerator. I grabbed a small yellow and red flowered glass from the counter and poured tap water in it for my grandmother.

Nonna came slowly into the kitchen. With each of her steps, the heel of her blue slippers clapped against the linoleum. Her feet dragged along as most of her weight concentrated on her upper body. Her arms quivered as she grasped the walker. She took a seat.

"Phoooo," she let out a sigh. Her bottom lip extended to let the relief escape her mouth.

I grabbed her walker and set it against the wall and then watched as my grandmother took a sip of water. Despite everything she was going through, she looked good. Her face was healthy and robust most days. She also seemed to be in better spirits since the telephone call.

I turned my gaze to view the yard from the screen door held open thanks to the hydraulic arm. For a summer day, the air was dry and the breeze was refreshing. The cicadas serenaded us as we sat and ate quietly. It was nice not to have to run to a doctor's appointment today.

No sooner had we sat down to eat when lunch was finished. I found myself at the kitchen sink for the second time in four hours. I rested my head against the white steel cabinet as I thoroughly washed each glass and small plate. I made sure my finger did not rub against the crack in one of the dishes.

Nonna walked slowly back to the bedroom. Normally at this time of the day she would pull out her gold-rimmed glasses, a far cry from the gray and black 'cat's eye' glasses she wore years ago, and read her Italian newsletters from various sanctuaries and organizations in Italy. There was one pamphlet in particular that always depicted the Virgin Mother holding the infant Jesus. Then there were the numerous saint cards, which she kept on her night table next to a green rosary—all within arm's length.

I turned and looked over my left shoulder and caught a glimpse of Nonna's blue slipper as it slid into the bedroom.

"How do you feel, Nonna?"

I waited for an answer, but all I heard was her walker stop. Then, as I stood above the sink with my head comfortably supported by the cabinet, I noticed she was heading my way.

"*Se Dio vuole.* If God a want," she started, her head looking down watching the veins in her hands enlarge as her grip grew tighter around the rubber handles of the walker. "I getta better."

She moved within a foot of me. The gap in our height was clearly evident. My brown eyes looked down at her as I tried to think of a reply. My blue tank top was spotted with water that had bounced off the bottom of the sink.

"Don't worry Nonna, you will," I said, believing my words.

"Come si dice?" (*How do you say?*) She was trying to find the word.

Her eyes looked upward as if trying to pull the word out of the air.

"Ahh." Her eyes lit up. *"Providenza!"* Her right hand pointed upward. Her hand placement was that of a statue of a saint. Her right hand's index finger pointed skyward, her thumb extended, and the rest of her fingers gently folded.

"Oh," I said. I turned off the running water and placed the last cup upside down on the rack. Taking the same hand towel I had used earlier, I wiped my hands dry then turned around to let my backside rest against the rim of the sink.

"You understandda?" Her eyes looked into my face for acknowledgement.

"Yes. Providence, whatever is God's will." Following Nonna's lead, my eyes turned upward to make the dramatic point.

"Si!" she said, looking at me approvingly. "God's a will."

She shuffled back into her bedroom. Her light blue, almost white housedress moved gracefully as she disappeared behind the doorway.

I stood there knowing this was a very different conversation from ones I normally had with Nonna. Something deep inside told me this was a special conversation. One that would transcend the small room and be remembered long after she was gone or I thought if we were lucky, once she got better. Most of all, it was a conversation only the two of us had taken part.

Despite the enormity of her illness and the daily pain and the struggle she endured, my grandmother was not ready to give up just yet. I understood what she meant. If she were to get better, it would have to be from divine intercession. She placed her life in God's hands, and hoped the saints to whom she prayed each and every day would assist her in this mission.

I heard Nonna sit on the bed and draw the covers about her legs. I stopped to reflect on my own weaknesses, which were many. I doubted I would have the same courage as she, despite the pain and loss of quality of life she was experiencing.

I stared down at my water-logged fingers as I folded the dishtowel and draped it neatly over the edge of the sink.

I heard the faint jingling of the rosary from the next room and smiled.

10

The News is Delivered

With the exception of the myriad of doctor appointments, which I soon found out were all for naught, the remainder of the summer was uneventful. However, I sensed deep within a change brewing, and that change was more than just the summer coming to an end.

My stomach carried a perpetual knot, and there was little in the way of happiness for me. Nobody spoke of any good news, for there was none. The absence of which grew heavy on my heart. My optimism was replaced with depression and it was starting to take a toll on my morale.

◆　　　◆　　　◆

The shockingly blue skies and refreshing breeze greeted the September day. With Nonna in the hospital for the past two days, there was nothing for Charles to do today except get his dad's signature on some hospital paperwork. A week earlier, Charles had decided to volunteer at the hospital and needed to return the authorization to the director of the program so he could start the following week.

"Wow," Charles exclaimed, as he exited the green and beige shingle house.

He took a deep breath of the cool, clean air. He was glad he made the decision to wear his light blue windbreaker. He would need it on his walk to the hospital, a distance of a mile or so from home. It was almost 11:30 in the morning and the sun had not yet warmed the air.

Tony, having taken the day off from work, left the house early to spend time by his mother's bedside. Charles' trip to the hospital would accomplish two things. He would obtain his dad's signature on the paperwork and see his grandmother.

Charles was volunteering time at the hospital with one of the few friends he had made in high school, a guy by the name of Roy. Roy was everything Charles was not. Roy was popular. Everyone in school knew who Roy was. But Charles was careful not to confuse being known with popularity.

Roy was the biggest freshman, not only in girth, but in personality. His voice echoed off the tiled walls of the school's corridor. You always knew when Roy was around. The one thing Charles liked about him was his upbeat disposition. Roy didn't seem to care what people said or thought about him. To Charles that was refreshing, especially since he had spent his life worrying about what people thought of him, and trying to obtain validation. Roy didn't need any of this.

Charles made his way past the security desk and up to the fourth floor. This was his grandmother's second admittance to the hospital in the past five months. The first one had been in May when she started receiving chemo. The doctors wanted to monitor her dosage and reaction, if any, to the medication. She had been on the same floor, but as Charles recalled in the very last room around the left bend of the corridor. Her bed was by the far wall in the small, mauve-painted room.

Nonna was in good spirits during that day in May when her grandson visited. She even joked with him when he showed up wearing black pants.

"Whyya you a wear blacka pants?" she asked her lanky grandson. "I'mma no dead yet."

Charles sat frozen, but she jokingly slapped his right knee. She laughed, but to him it was no laughing matter.

This time Charles was afraid this was it. The past few days had been tumultuous ones. Especially difficult was the news Nonna received on September 12. Tony, Josephine and Diego told their mother she was fighting cancer.

◆   ◆   ◆

The roar of the train passing above on the elevated tracks could be heard from four blocks away as my father and I crossed busy Grand Avenue. The late evening provided a respite from the glaring sun. The colors in the sky provided a nice contrast to the green trees that lined the street. Deep pink swatches, as if created by a master painter, crisscrossed the sky like a canvas.

"We told Nonna she has cancer." My father's words struck me as if I had been hit by one of the many cars that whizzed by.

All I could do was look at him quizzically. But he was oblivious to the stare, and continued walking. His face showed signs of worry. His forehead creased, his eyes, thin slits.

"You mean she didn't know all this time? I can't believe she didn't know. What did she think she had with all the pain?" I was incredulous as I quizzed my dad.

"A virus," he responded quietly. "She thought she had a virus."

Dad had just finished his sentence when an older woman passed us going in the opposite direction. Her cascading gray hair fell lightly on the black shoulders of her dress. She yelled in Greek for her young grandson to wait. Her arms waved excitedly. The three gold bracelets on her right wrist jingled and rolled down to the middle of her arm.

A whiff of souvlaki grilling and sizzling on a street vendor's cart we had just passed caught my attention. I realized how hungry I was.

"I tell you, Charlie," my father continued. "It's such a relief to have told her."

His words sounded different. The change was visible. I could tell. Behind the clear frames of my dad's glasses, I could see relief in his eyes. It was as if the weight of the world had been lifted from his shoulders. I glanced in his direction. He was still pensive, but his face appeared calm and relaxed with the exception of the perpetual crevices running the length of his forehead. I noticed the dark hair just above my dad's ears was starting to turn gray. I still could not believe that all this time Nonna had absolutely no idea her pain was the sign of something that she would not recover from.

"Was she in denial or just ignorant?" I thought to myself.

A few weeks later, I was yet again surprised. I was told Nonna had selected her headstone, a depiction of the Sacred Heart of Jesus.

The reality that she knew she was dying hurt me more than anything.

11

The Fight is Over

The elevator hesitated at the fourth floor before the doors opened to loud moaning from one of the rooms along the corridor.

Two ladies walked gingerly along the hallway. As I passed I heard one say, "Poor thing," in a hushed voice. One was prisoner to a wheeled silver pole with a clear glucose bag hanging from it. IV tubes snaked down to her thin and frail hands.

The shorter of the women shook her wrinkly face in response to the comment. "Aiiiiii. Aiiiiii."

The moaning grew as I got closer to Nonna's room. My stomach went into overdrive as if I had just come through two huge loops of a roller coaster. I was dreading to find out where these agonizing sounds originated. It soon became all too clear. Upon entering Room 409 my fears were confirmed.

The bed closest to the door was empty. Against the sunlit window, I saw my dad's silhouette. He was leaning against the radiator, his left arm up as if supporting his face. He wore his glasses. His lips pouted.

As I walked inside, Nonna's bed came into view behind the partially closed, striped curtain. Drawing closer still, I saw her hands lying along her sides. The bed was propped up to about a thirty-degree angle.

Her face was hidden behind a green transparent oxygen mask. She moaned with every breath, each painful exhale evenly spaced. I stood at the foot of the bed absorbing the scene.

Her hair fanned about her face was pulled down around her ears by the elastic cord holding the mask in place. I noticed how remarkably young she appeared. There were very few wrinkles to speak of and her face actually seemed to glow.

"What are you doing today?" my dad asked me in a hushed voice.

"Oh, I just need you to sign these papers so I can take them down to the volunteer department."

I removed the papers from the pocket of my jeans and unfolded them for my dad to sign.

My grandmother opened her eyes, be it ever so brief, at the sound of my voice. Her trusted companion and helper during the last several months had returned. She had probably heard my voice, but was too weak and in too much pain to do anything more than signal with her eyes recognition of my presence.

"God, how did she get this bad in so short a time?" I pondered as my dry fingers rubbed my eyes. She had gone from bad to worse, her condition graver than when my sister and I had visited just two days earlier.

◆   ◆   ◆

It was a blessing the teachers at the high school were still on strike. If not for the walkout, I would have been sitting in some classroom today. But this bright and warm Wednesday was full of promise. The birds chirped from the peach tree in our backyard and nibbled on the bread my father had scattered on the cinder block walkway leading past the fig trees and waist-high tomato plants.

With not much else to do, I figured I would make a visit to St. Patrick's, this time with my sister, Maria. Being a year younger and just beginning her freshman year in the same school as me, she was also free because of the strike.

Besides lighting candles and praying to the likeness of St. Anthony, we made a point of stopping by the gift shop just inside the church where I purchased a small, six-inch plastic statue of Saint Theresa, the Little Flower. I knew this would make a nice addition to my growing collection. Our day ended with a visit to Nonna.

The all too familiar ping of the elevator signaled our arrival at the fourth floor. We exited the elevator to the right and my sister and I walked along the narrow corridor to Nonna's room. Lucky for Nonna she was still the only occupant. My sneakers grabbed the highly-glossed tiles as I entered on my tiptoes. We found Nonna sleeping, but she wasn't the only one in the darkened room.

Aunt Concettina was by her side, as she had been for a majority of Nonna's entire hospital stay. Concettina was very much like her half-sister lying in the bed. She was small in stature, but large in kindness. Curly brown hair circled her face softened by her plump cheeks. All one needed to do to know what she was thinking was look at her eyes. She wore a black skirt with a multi-colored striped knitted shirt that clung close to her frame.

I placed the brown bag containing the statue of Saint Theresa at the foot of Nonna's bed. I noticed in the dim light that Nonna's breathing came in waves.

Her chest heaved up with each intake of oxygen. With every exhale, her face showed the pain and difficulty of keeping up this basic, life-sustaining activity. Each exhale was accompanied by a light moan. I could hear the congestion building in her lungs.

I stood at the foot of the bed and looked at her under the stark white sheets. Her gray black hair was fanned out on the pillow above her smooth and unblemished face. Her arms, speckled with little red blood spots from needles, were exposed above the bed sheets. My eyes continued their journey down to her hands and fingernails.

"Shit!" I thought to myself, fixated on Nonna's nails. I recalled a conversation my sister and I had with our friend Susan just a week earlier. She had basically told us that you could tell if a person was dying by their fingernails. If they were blue, it meant that the end was near.

Nonna's were blue.

"Has she been sleeping long, Aunt Concettina?" I asked.

"No, juussta a few minuttsa," she said solemnly. Pensive, her open right hand never moved from her cheek.

My mind wandered to happier times, Nonna and her sister's laughing and chatting at the long, well stocked dinner table.

I felt my chest and throat tighten and I sighed.

"Maria, you go with you brother…" my aunt continued to speak just as I saw Nonna's eyes flutter awake. It took her a good minute to get oriented before she recognized me standing about seven feet away. She gave a weak smile, but it lit up her face and mine.

I moved to the cold railing and kissed her. Like the bars, she too felt cold.

"Concettina," Nonna said, looking at her sister. "Aqua."

My aunt heeded her request for water. Nonna's tongue patted her lips trying to moisten them. Concettina had finished pouring the water from its bland yellow pitcher into a very small cup. With her right hand, my aunt lifted Nonna's head and held it slightly above the pillow to allow my grandmother to drink. Her greasy hair lay limp on the pillow.

My grandmother was pleased. It had come to this. Being happy with something as insignificant as a small cup of water. I didn't want her to be happy with just this. I wanted her to be happy like when she had the family over and made homemade pizza or pasta, which she did so adeptly. I wanted back those Sundays sitting outside on her back stoop sipping a cup of coffee. I didn't want her to go away.

"Hello, Mrs. Alaimo," a booming voice from behind startled the heck out of us. The small room was crowded as a doctor now joined the four of us. He wasn't a doctor I had seen before; tall and relatively young with a bushy mustache that separated his thin lips and beaky nose. He greeted the group as he went about the business taking Nonna's vitals.

I moved out of the way allowing him access to her pulse and studied the doctor's face intently. It finally dawned on me that this was Nonna's oncologist, the one who had his office on Crescent Street right up the block from here, the one with the turquoise-colored door.

"How do you feel, Mrs. Alaimo?" he asked, as his right forefinger bore down on her wrist. It was a rhetorical question. He seemed not to care about a response.

Nonna had suffered a seizure the afternoon before. With her head at a strange angle, she found it difficult to respond. She was also a bit groggy from being aroused from her midday nap. Her tired eyes watched the foot of the bed and then moved to me. Her face was somewhat gray. Her response to the doctor was inaudible as she fought to catch her breath.

"Che Maria?" (*What Maria?*) Concettina leaned over to make out what Nonna was saying.

"Dice a dottore," Nonna looked at me as she spoke, her voice pleading. *"Che Io voglio morire, non voglio soffrire."*

Her request drove a knife through my heart.

"No!" I quickly responded to her request. This was probably the one and only time I had ever said this word to Nonna.

"Maria?" Concettina bit her bottom lip, held back tears and looked at me. My sister standing to my left was oblivious to what our grandmother had just asked.

"What did she say?" the physician looked to me waiting for an answer.

Put on the spot, I answered without looking at him.

"She asked me to tell you that she wants to die." My eyes never left my sneakers. "She does not want to suffer anymore."

"Now, now, Mrs. Alaimo, don't worry," he said, but in my opinion doing a tremendously poor job in his attempt to comfort her. He seemed to brush her comment aside.

My grandmother had given up faith that she would get well.

"What kind of pain was she in that would make her say something like that?" I asked myself.

My hands, which I held behind my back the entire time to support me against the wall, were quickly becoming numb.

Before I knew it, I realized we had been there for well over an hour. I quickly exited the room to use the bathroom. I wanted to be sure I was okay for the walk home.

I returned to the room just in time to find Nonna removing the statue I had purchased from its colorful box. She immediately kissed the saint's yellow painted gown.

"Ciali, questa e per me?" she asked, questioning if the statue was for her.

"Yes, Nonna," I responded, not having the heart to say no.

She kissed the statue once more and handed it to Concettina who placed it on the bed stand. Although I was disappointed, I knew she needed the statue more than I did right now, and it brought me a sense of comfort that this little gift buoyed her spirits.

Before leaving I hesitated. I didn't know if I would ever see my grandmother alive again. I stood motionless once more at the foot of the bed and looked at the person who had become the center of my life. For me, everything revolved around her. Unfortunately, it had only been the last few years that I had grown close to her.

I took a deep breath and wished that while I was growing up I had spent more time with her. There were so many times when my parents had events and I refused to stay with her, opting to stay with Aunt Concettina and my cousins instead. Nonna always had nice things in her house, the one on Thirty-sixth Street, and I felt uncomfortable there at times.

When my siblings and I were growing up, Nonna had lived right up the block from us on Fourteenth Street in Astoria. I was young and spent many days there walking up the block from our home to her house by the public library to spend time with her.

I chuckled inside as I thought of all those times I did not want to go to school—kindergarten at the time. On Sundays when we were visiting, I would go into Nonna's kitchen and feign illness, spitting onto my index finger and putting the liquid near my eyes to make it appear as if I had been crying.

"God, I can't believe that of all the things I might recall about her, these were my memories," I thought to myself.

Nonna was always there for me. She always came to my defense and supported me. Now, ten years later, I was the one who had become her comforter and supporter.

◆   ◆   ◆

"How is she?" I asked, realizing how stupid a question it was the moment it left my lips. It was evident she was not doing well at all.

My father did not respond, but rather shrugged his shoulders as he handed me back the signed hospital authorization forms. I immediately and indifferently stuffed them into the inside pocket of my blue waist-length jacket.

Nonna had suffered two morphine-induced seizures that week. My grandfather had been so upset that he had chased a nurse out of the room and down the hall, yelling and waving his crutch at her. A priest had been called to administer the last rites.

Despite the abundance of natural sunlight from the windows to the right of Nonna's bed, the room was rather dark and easy on the eyes.

Life was going on all around us; people laughing and talking, the quick burst of a car horn from the street below, a gentleman coming out of the pizzeria across the way with a hot slice in his hand.

"It is miserably unfair," I thought. "Up until just a year ago, it seemed Nonna was really doing well. Now this."

For some reason I thought of all those walks just a couple years ago that Nonna and I had taken to pick Josephine up from the pastry shop where she had worked. On the nights when I slept over, we went to pick her up. I had a bad habit of constantly turning around when I walked with Nonna, which she was quick to point out. She would always hit me, jokingly of course, to get me to stop. We never waited for Josephine right in front of the store, but off to the side just a few doors down. Nonna didn't want to infringe on her daughter's space. She was pretty cool about things like that.

With a deep sigh and a heavy heart, I went to the right side of Nonna's bed and patted her right hand lightly.

"Bye, Nonna," I said. My polyester jacket swooshed as I brought my hand to my face and brushed my hair from my eyes. I leaned over and kissed her cheek, careful not to disturb the mask encircling her mouth and nose. The oxygen mask brushed against the right side of my smooth, hairless face. She opened her eyes briefly. No smile this time. I took one final moment by her bedside, stood expressionless, and watched as she fought to breathe. With each inhalation she grimaced and cried.

I was upset at what this illness was doing to her. Nonna did not deserve this at all. She was nothing but good and kind, but the disease treated her savagely.

While upset over this, I was even angrier she was leaving at a time when I was getting to really know her and truly appreciate her value to me.

I had a lot more living to do and I wanted her to be there to witness the high points of my life—after having gone through all the shit I had been through the last year. But it was not meant to be.

"Bye, Nonna," I whispered again, and touched her arm just above the bed sheet. I gazed at her one final time, and like those summer days I spent memorizing her features and the sound of her voice, I studied her this time too. I felt I would soon need all those memories. I left the room not fully realizing this was the last time I would see her alive.

12

September 19, 1981

Although I was awake lying in my bed, the harsh, tinny, lifeless sound of the doorbell startled me. Its echo chimed coldly through the house on that gray Saturday morning seeming to forewarn us of the news waiting on the other side of the door.

I could discern through my open bedroom door my mother donning her slippers and going to the front door, her feet slapping against the linoleum. The same slapping sound I heard when she awoke every morning at three o'clock to check on us in our beds.

"Just making sure you're breathing," she would tell us the next morning. Thanks to her early morning walks, I was never able to get an uninterrupted night's sleep.

My father was at the door. I hadn't realized he had not returned home from the hospital the night before. The sun shone dimly through the morning clouds, the early light glowing through the large metal slats of the blinds.

"How is everything?" I heard my mom ask. She closed the heavy wooden door. The click of the lock echoed through the foyer.

There was a brief pause before my dad responded.

"She died."

Like the air out of a balloon, my father sighed and cried at the same time. He had been holding it in for some time. Up until today, this was the first time I had ever seen or heard him cry.

Instinctually, or perhaps to announce the news to someone who had not heard it, I jumped out of bed and shook my brother who was still asleep in his bed on the other side of the room.

"Wake up, Mark. Nonna died!" I headed out of the room before my younger sibling even had a chance to respond. I watched my father who was seated at the dining room table. My mother walked over and placed a hot cup of coffee in front of him. I joined him sitting directly across at the other end of the oblong table.

"So, she died?" I asked. I thought it odd the words came out with no great emotion. I wasn't even crying.

My mom reached in the cupboard, pulled out a mug and filled it up with the dark, rich brew. Even at my age I loved the smell of coffee brewing. She placed the mug in front of me. There were questions I wanted answered so I started with the first of many.

"So how did she die?" I asked. "What time?"

Dad took a long sip before beginning to recount the last moments for us.

"She died around five this morning," he began. "And everyone was there. We called Aunt Antonia Alaimo and Brucculeri, and Aunt Concettina. They were all there. Josephine and Diego, too. We knew it was going to be the end." He stopped and sipped.

Following his lead, I brought the cup to my lips and took a long slow sip of my coffee allowing the warm elixir to waken my system.

"The hospital was good about letting us all stay in the room. Luckily, they never put anyone else in the bed next to hers," he continued, his face ashen.

"Was she in pain?" I asked inquisitively.

"She got worse through the night. She was screaming loudly at times."

I recalled how Nonna looked and sounded when I saw her yesterday afternoon. My father continued to tell us how the pain enveloped her whole body. She shook violently as the fatal disease consumed every last cell. After this enormous amount of pain, there was no more pain to be felt. The disease had finally burned itself out.

"It was around two this morning when she seemed to rest." My father stopped and stared ahead. His fingers tapped the white ceramic cup that kept his hands warm. I was so consumed by the story I had hardly touched my now lukewarm coffee.

"Nonna started calling for Diego," continued my father. "Diego kept saying, 'Mom I'm right here,' but Nonna told him to be quiet." A slight smile crossed Dad's face. "She wasn't calling him, Nonna said, but my other brother." (this was my father's younger brother also named Diego who died at the age of one).

What my father told me next was unbelievable.

"After a while she got up and walked around," he continued.

I stared in amazement. "What?" I half muttered.

"There was no pain, no sign that anything was wrong."

After not being able to walk unassisted for more than seven months Nonna actually got up out of bed and walked the room! Divine intercession had given her the opportunity to walk the earth one last time.

"It was just a few minutes after that when she started going in and out of sleep." My father lifted his coffee and sipped. He spoke into his cup. "She called for Diego again, and then she said that Padre Pio was at Immaculate Conception."

I leaned forward in my chair waiting for his next words, my feet propped on the chair across from me.

Just then I realized Maria and Mark were still asleep in their rooms.

Immaculate Conception had been Nonna's parish. It's a beautiful open church with life-size statues of saints scattered throughout. Nonna's favorite was the Pieta. I could only recount a handful of times when I had accompanied my grandmother to church just to drop in and light one of the many candles in front of the statue, the candles' red glass holder flickering in an electronic dance.

After kneeling and saying a prayer Nonna would stand up on the cushioned kneeler and with her left hand, grasp the brick railing, lean and touch the clothed knee of the Blessed Mother, and then her son Jesus who lay in her arms. Then reaching her hand to her mouth, Nonna kissed the forefinger of her clasped hand. It was such an Italian thing to do. With so many others repeating the ritual, the Blessed Mother's blue robe was worn to a yellowish, white around her bended knee.

"Padre Pio was at Immaculate Conception," I repeated my dad's words trying to picture Nonna saying them.

Nonna admired and prayed often to Padre Pio, the Capuchin monk who was blessed with the stigmata of Christ. In her night table drawer, Nonna kept a number of Padre Pio's prayer cards alongside her green stone rosary. She said the rosary each day, her fingers gliding along the smooth glass beads. She used them so often that some of the metal clasps, which kept each bead in alignment, had become worn. To keep the row of emerald beads connected to the silver crucifix, she had repaired them with thread.

Between frequent sips of coffee, my father told us that about five ten that morning with her family around her, Nonna started going in and out of consciousness.

"It was during these moments where she kept saying that she had to cross the water and climb the stairs. The Blessed Mother was at the top of the stairs with the baby Jesus. She said she needed to cross the water to get to the stairs," my father uttered once more in a hushed, pensive whisper. "That was the last time. She closed her eyes and that was it. She died. The time was five ten."

I was upset with myself for a number of reasons. The first not being able to cry, and I also had a deep regret that I had not been there to say goodbye to my grandmother one last time.

Having taken care of her for so many months I missed the most important event, the culmination or climax if you will, of my grandmother's illness. Instead, I chose to spend the day seeing a movie with my sister. I sat there at the table and continued to regret my decision of the day before.

Something wasn't registering with me. There was still an element of disbelief that Nonna was truly gone. To me, she was still lying in bed at the hospital. I would put on my sneakers and visit her in an instant. But a visit that day would have been to no avail.

Emerging from the bathroom, I found Mark sitting at the table crying a bit. He was only eleven-years-old, and I questioned why he was crying and I wasn't. I grew more frustrated with myself as I retired to my bedroom to get dressed.

My dad was going to see Grandpa and I considered accompanying him, though a sense of urgency was lacking. I moved halfheartedly as I slid into my jeans, not knowing whether to go or not. But my father seemed worried and I decided to go with him.

I headed out the back door and took a seat in the striped canvas chair having just finished putting on my clothes and a thick white sweater to keep away the chill of early morning.

My eyes stared toward the house and then up to the pitched roof. A cold breeze crossed my face. My nose was cold. I pressed my hands deep into the pockets of my white cotton sweater. The door slammed and Dad came into the backyard and joined me.

We walked the short block practically without saying a word. Upon reaching Nonna's house, I climbed the stairs and held the railing where only days before she had held it. It was difficult to think of Nonna in the past tense. If I had one wish it would be to turn back time, even just a few hours so I could be at the hospital with her and tell her that I loved her and would never forget her.

Nonno let my father and me in. His face was thin. He had started cleaning up the second floor apartment. His tenants had moved out only one month ago. They were a friendly, elderly couple who had lived there for a few years. Their name escaped me at the moment. The gentleman was always smartly dressed but balding. The hair he did have was red. His wife was pleasant, too.

"Mr. Klein!" I finally remembered their name.

On holidays, the Klein's were always treated to a plate of Nonna's special meals—homemade manicotti, perhaps meatballs.

◆   ◆   ◆

Those pre-holiday evenings were special for me. Before Easter or Thanksgiving, I always tried to sleep at Nonna's so I could help her the next day. In the basement, the stark white metal sink, oven, and refrigerator became the center of activity for lots of prep work.

Nonna kept all the tools she needed for a fantastic holiday meal in the shelves lining the wall and storeroom of her basement. Her specialty was homemade manicotti, which I had helped her make on many a holiday. Those pre-holiday evenings always started the same way. She would reach into the white cabinets and pull out a roll of aluminum foil. The cabinets always made a tinny sound when the magnet on the door met with the metal of the frame.

Nonna would cut the aluminum foil into five-inch by five-inch squares, about thirty of them. Having already prepared the crepe batter (for the manicotti), she would heat a small fry pan and with a ladle, drop in a bit of batter and flip the crepe over at just the right time. She would put each crepe between pieces of foil, and then I would take the tower of crepes and place them in the front room of the basement where they stayed overnight.

Although a basement, the room was cozy with a couch and a comfy chair and a television and full bathroom. (It was the only bathroom in the house until Nonna got sick and Nonno built one on the main floor.) The centerpiece in the room was the large dining table. On all sides the table was graced with low back, white and brown Formica chairs.

Adorning one wall right above a little closet underneath the staircase hung a picture of the Blessed Mother represented as Our Lady of Sorrows. Her face and eyes downcast. Her dark blue robe covered her head, her hand clasping the robe at her neck. It was a beautiful picture in a simple frame. For me, this picture was the focal point of the stark white walls.

◆   ◆   ◆

I sat in the entry to the second floor apartment taking a seat on the third step from the bottom. I reached my left arm to gently grasp the glass knob of the door. My fingers encircled the large clear cabochon. I stared through the nine-pane glass door. After hearing banging coming from upstairs I finally got up quite lazily and climbed the short staircase. I found my grandfather in the front room on his wooden ladder. My father was handing him tiles. They were retiling the ceiling. The double windows in the room were bare and thanks to the western exposure, allowed an abundance of natural light to come into the tiny three-room abode. At this hour of the day, eleven in the morning, the sun was not quite yet overhead. Leaning against the wide window frame I looked out and saw high clouds slowly enveloping the blue sky. Nonno left the room briefly and I turned to my father.

"Why is he doing this now?" my voice angry. "God, Nonna just died and he's worried about doing this!"

"Charlie, he needs to keep his mind busy," my father said patiently.

Starting for the doorway I shot back, "I just think it's ridiculous."

I left the room and headed down the staircase taking a seat on the same step I had rested on earlier. I was trying to make sense of the whole day, trying to make sense of what had happened and trying to let it register that I had lost someone very close to me. I was so unsure about how I should act since I never had someone die on me. However, I knew you don't put up ceiling tiles.

Five and one half hours had passed since Nonna's death.

Time distanced me from her. Whenever my eyes came upon a clock I looked at it and calculated how many hours had passed since Nonna had died. I missed her. That gap between Nonna and the rest of the family was growing by the minute. I lost count of how many times I wished that time would be turned back to that moment she passed away. I wished I had been at the hospital. Out of everyone who should have been there I should have been. After all, I had taken good care of her those last months helping her around the house or just keeping her company.

I walked down to the kitchen and sat there, my head rested on my right hand as I gazed out the window. Looking to my left, my eyes came upon the bed she was never going to rest in again. Her bedside had become a central point of discussion during those last months when she was not able to rise. There were many times when my father and I visited and just sat by her bed. Those visits often shifted to the topic of me getting a job.

◆   ◆   ◆

It was another walk after dinner.
The date was August 14, 1981.

Charles missed the autumn darkness of the night on his walk this evening. Being mid-August, the sun was still out in full force as he entered the house to find Nonna in her bedroom.

"Hey Nonna," he greeted her from the sunlit kitchen.

She was wearing her glasses and reading one of her many Italian religious magazines. Charles grabbed a chair from the kitchen and headed into her room careful not to bump the chair into the foot of the bed. Charles, by this time quite tall, bent over and kissed her. His father was right behind him, chair in hand as well.

Her room was darker than the kitchen because the curtains were drawn. The faint light from the kitchen illuminated the black handle of the phone and worked illumination wonders on the small blue bottle of Brioschi that kept her rosary and saint cards company on her nightstand.

Most of the time only Charles and his dad chatted in the room. Nonno, opting not to participate, often remained in the backyard. Nonna always appeared to look very comfortable propped up against three large fluffy pillows.

She faced the kitchen, and to her right she could see through the doors to the living room. Her intricately woven flowered bedspread was always wrapped and tucked neatly just above her waist and folded over once. Her arms lay atop the cottony crease.

The early evening sky would slowly turn dark while the trio sat and chatted; sometimes in English and at times, when Tony and his mother decided, in Sicilian. The cool evening breeze blew softly across the yard through one of the opened windows and cooled them off. They rarely used the fan bolted into the other window of the room.

Visiting Nonna made Charles feel as if he was making a daily spiritual journey, almost akin to climbing a Tibetan mountain to listen to the Dalai Lama or a wise sage. This was especially true when Nonna imparted her wishes for him. Most of the time it centered on him finding a job.

"Go a La Guli," she often told her grandson, referring him to the well-known pastry shop in their area. "Tell themma thata Giuseppina izza you zia (aunt)."

"Okay, Nonna. Okay."

With everything going on that summer, Charles never did get a chance to apply for a position at the pastry shop.

◆　　　◆　　　◆

The remainder of that gray, September day was a blur. Besides performing the most mundane of tasks, I had an insatiable need to go through old family photos. When my family had met up at my grandparent's house, my sister and I took the opportunity to break away to the basement to see what treasures could be found in the cobalt blue tin that once held Danish butter cookies.

I made my way down the short flight of stairs and slid open the brown closet doors to reveal the time capsule waiting on the top shelf. I placed the round cookie tin on the dining table. This was the same table where I had watched Nonna make pasta so many times before, the same table where we had eaten so many meals as a family. A plastic covering protected the lace tablecloth.

Twelve hours had passed since Nonna died.

My sister joined me as we sorted through the small pile of gems. Memories long forgotten. We must have sat there for an hour pouring over old family pictures taken at a variety of functions. One photo taken in my grandmother's backyard showed the entire family gathered around the stoop during one of the many barbeques. I wrinkled my nose and could actually smell sweet sausage sizzling on the grill. It was the thin kind of sausage without the fennel—the type I liked best. The pictures with Nonna were especially valuable to me. These ordinary, everyday photos became priceless.

Our treasure hunt was short-lived when my mother called down the stairs to my sister.

"We're going Maria."

Thirteen hours had passed now.

Placing the photos in the perfectly round tin, I headed up the stairs right behind Maria. I didn't feel like being in the basement alone. As we emerged through the narrow doorway, I saw my dad put on his coat. Josephine was there as well having just returned from the funeral parlor after selecting the dress that Nonna would wear and delivering it to the funeral home. She chose the purple gown Nonna had worn to Josephine's wedding a year earlier.

My family prepared to leave. However, I was to remain behind. The group gathered in the small kitchen and proceeded down the hall toward the door. Much to my dismay, my father had instructed me earlier that I was to sleep over at Nonno's house.

Now that everyone was leaving I resented my father for ordering me to do this. I had never thought twice about sleeping over when Nonna was there, but I was not especially close to my grandfather and dreaded having to be alone with him. To me, my grandfather was always angry. At what or with whom I never knew. My dad was concerned his father might have a difficult first night.

With everyone having left the house, I became acutely aware of my loneliness and the void that now existed. It was just Nonno and me. I didn't have the energy to do much but sit on the loveseat and stare aimlessly at the blank television screen. The whole day had passed, and I hadn't shed a single tear. It was just too hard for me to imagine she was gone.

This was the first time in my life I had lost someone so close, and perhaps I didn't believe it yet. I was in denial. Since I hadn't seen her die, in my head she was still alive and laying in that nondescript hospital bed. Even Nonno reacted indifferently as if nothing had changed. He wasn't crying either, although he was a bit nastier than usual.

Sixteen hours and fifteen minutes had passed since Nonna died.

I pushed the ornate coffee table out of the way making sure the glass candy dish centered on the inlaid white marble top did not tip over. I expertly removed the pillow cushion on the loveseat revealing the dark black frame and handle. I lifted the handle and pulled out the bed and quickly made it with the sheets Nonna always had ready for me whenever I slept over.

"Good night, Nonno," I yelled into the other dark room beyond the double doors. The only light on in the house was the one in the living room next to the sofa. I refused to shut it off. The white and gold lamp cast a bright glow onto the semi-gloss paint of the room. I hated the light, but I hated darkness more.

My grandfather had already tucked himself into bed. A grunt was the only recognition I heard from him. Finally, I hesitantly reached over to the lamp, but stopped before pushing the thin black rod that would send the room into total darkness. I heard Dad's voice in my head telling me as he often did, "The night is for the wolves." He loved repeating this old Sicilian saying to his kids.

I wasn't afraid so much of what the night held, but what the darkness represented; the end of the day. I didn't want this day to end, the first ever without Nonna. If I left the light on much longer I knew Nonno would say something. Having no choice, I gave in and clicked the black button.

I found my way under the thin sheet and brought it up to my nose as I often did. Although her light dimmed on this day, it would remain forever alive in my heart. This day was the defining moment in my life, and much like a picture develops in a darkroom, this night would be emblazoned in my memory and heart and would shape the person I would become.

It would take my eyes a few minutes to adjust to the dark. In the meantime, I lay on my back thinking about how I didn't want to be here right now. There was no way I was going to sleep easy. The house just wasn't the same without Nonna. Ever so faintly the ceiling started to come into view as my eyes became accustomed to the dark. Just a few hours earlier I had sat in this chair, which was now a very comfortable sofa bed. From this vantage point I watched the activity in the house. I saw my family coming and going. The phone calls, my aunt and father going to make the funeral arrangements and picking the clothes Nonna was going to wear. All I did was mark on a small calendar from the local bank, "Nonna Died," in the square that read September 19. It was hard to imagine that only a few days ago Nonna had been in this house. Now she was gone.

In all the years I had slept over, I never did get comfortable with the fact that everyone in this house always went to sleep at the same time. It was quite different coming from an environment where my dad usually went to bed first, followed by me. My mother and sister on the other hand, were sometimes up all night; the sounds of the television emanating from the living room comforting me. I needed noise to sleep. I needed to know there were people still awake.

Tonight found me once again a prisoner of the darkness and the abyss of silence. The streetlights glowing through the Venetian blinds behind my sofa bed played eerily with the porcelain horse vase that stood atop the stereo credenza. The shadows flickered and danced against the wall, while outside the gently swaying trees moved in the late night breeze. Headlights from an occasional passing car added to the ballet.

I finally dozed off, although not for long, perhaps an hour at best. I awoke laying on my right side, opened my eyes and gazed at the arm of the loveseat. I could feel my hot breath encircle my face. With only an inch separating my mouth from the arm of the chair there was little space for my exhalations. But something was different. My eyes were drawn to an area just above the golden upholstery.

Something or someone was there.

"Could it be?" I thought to myself. Not moving my body, I closed my eyes hard and reopened them. My heart raced and thumped through my thin cotton white undershirt.

Nonna stood in the doorway of the living room. I could clearly make out her upper body; the rest, hazy and shrouded in light mist. "The kind you get with dry ice," I thought. She was dressed in the purple gown. The beads on the bodice shimmered like twinkling stars. Her hair was perfectly coiffed. She was smiling. She was still here, it was no dream!

I must have swallowed hard because I could feel my throat hurt. I closed my eyes. "Surely the shadows are playing tricks," I thought, too paralyzed to speak. I worried my grief was getting the best of me. I opened my eyes. She was still there.

I propped my head up with my right arm and looked intently.

"It is her! It really is Nonna!" I thought.

I studied each part of her image. The details were too perfect to be anything but real. I paid careful attention to her hands. Their position struck me as odd. They were perfectly clasped. Her fingers remained side by side and formed a semi-circle, each hand fitting into the other like a piece of a puzzle. The back of her right hand faced upward, while her left hand was underneath; it's back facing the floor. The fingers on each hand never intertwined with the others.

She began moving ever so slowly to where I lay. I was unable to move. Everything below her hands and waist was shrouded in fog and her feet were not discernable. The mist surrounding her had taken on a beautiful warm glow, as if light was emanating from behind her. She floated toward me, all the while never moving her head or changing the smile on her face.

By the time she reached the loveseat, she was smiling at me, a smile I had never seen before. I returned her smile. She did not show any teeth. Her lips were together like Mona Lisa. However, for me the message was in her eyes. They conveyed her feelings. Looking into them I felt an incredible sense of love and peace. "Peaceful and calm within me," I would later recount. We looked at one another for perhaps five seconds, then as fast as she had appeared, she was gone. I remained propped up on my elbow wondering if what I had witnessed was real.

"How could I imagine this?" I said aloud. A bead of sweat dripped from my forehead and down onto my bare arm. I looked over to the front windows. I became aware that my heart was resuming its normal rhythm once again. "How could I imagine such detail?"

With a sigh of wonder and a feeling that something utterly and truly amazing had occurred, I plopped my head back onto the thin pillow. She must have read my thoughts. I had felt guilty, sad, and depressed about not having the chance to say goodbye, and never having the opportunity to tell her just how much I loved her and what she meant to me. How she forever changed my life through the lessons I learned from her, and how her struggle to fight the disease that ultimately consumed her body never touched who she was. I admired her spirituality, courage, and faith in God, all of which could not be destroyed.

"Perhaps she came to me to thank me for taking care of her all those months and never questioning, but always prepared to do whatever needed to be done to make her day a bit better," I thought. "Whatever the reason, she visited me." This much I knew.

I fell asleep thinking about the morning, eager to tell everyone about Nonna's visit. "Nobody is going to believe me," I whispered secretly to myself as my eyelids grew weak. And nobody did.

13

The Wake

We parked in the rear of the white stucco, tile roofed building. The high wrought iron gate around the structure made the place resemble an Italian villa like the ones found along Lake Como.

The facade showed signs of aging and neglect. There were areas where the yellow stucco was faded. In other places the paint was peeling away exposing brick just below the thin topcoat.

I bolted from the blue Pontiac Ventura, brushed the hair from my eyes, straightened my black windbreaker and started walking. Patience was not one of my strong suits and waiting on my parents, not an option. My sister Maria joined me on the short walk around the corner, a good twenty paces ahead of our parents and younger brother.

The wind whipped up the dead leaves, coaxing them back to life after forcing them from their perch high atop the giant oak trees lining the street. The dried leaves swirled in circles crackling their discontent, some refusing to be hoisted by the breeze. Many of the newly fallen were still cloaked in the vibrant colors of fall. They were not yet brittle and brown as their ancestors. They fluttered, skipped, swirled and turned as they danced in the wind. Their vibrant colors made them appear alive, a sharp contrast to the monotone canopy of the colorless and somber sky.

I walked through the chaotic maelstrom of the once verdant foliage. But much like the leaves that lined my path, I was powerless against the recent events that fate had placed upon me.

My mood on this, the first day of my grandmother's wake, was much like the rather nondescript day. I carried myself well for a young man of fifteen, a direct result of my experiences over the past year.

This was my first wake and I didn't quite know how I should act. Despite the fact that I had no point of reference, I thought I looked the part without trying all that hard. Outwardly, the contrast between my young face and the deep-set baggy eyes signaled how this death had affected me.

Inward I was devoid of feeling. Not a numbness, for surely I would have known if that was the case. This was a feeling of nothingness. No sadness. No joy. Nothing except perhaps discomfort from the tightness of the waistband from my pants as it dug into my plump abdomen.

I turned left past the high-scrolled gate, and was the first to reach the forest green door. It was locked. I searched for the bell, found it and pressed hard, taking out my anger on the white button. I stretched my legs and with both of my palms set flat against the wood paneling of the door, I leaned forward standing on the tips of my black lace-up shoes and peered in through the three square panes of glass lining the top of the entranceway. The view was straight down a hallway to the entrance of the first floor viewing room to the left of the corridor.

I strained my neck and caught a glimpse of Nonna. She lay at the far end crowning the long narrow viewing room. She was all alone waiting for her family to come and visit her one last time. Time seemed to stand still as I looked in through the window. I took in the moment and tried to memorize the scene reminiscent of the countless times I had waited for Nonna to answer the door, the latest just a few weeks ago. This time I knew Nonna would not be opening the door. She was sublimely radiant waiting expectantly for her family and visitors. She appeared shrouded in fog. Her hair nicely done, rested on a small pillow.

From the corner of my eye, a portly man appeared from a back room. His rotund body and shiny head adorned with a pair of glasses came toward the door.

I was no longer alone. The entire family was gathered behind me. Mark stood quietly in his brown pants and beige jacket. He looked awfully thin alongside Mom. Our brood of five stood silently while just beyond the tall gates and shrubs life continued as usual. The small front garden of the funeral parlor provided some seclusion from the commotion going on all around us, but we could hear cars and buses zooming past in either direction along busy Grand Avenue.

I glanced across the street toward the front of the beige brick apartment building. A few kids, some still dressed in shorts, played hopscotch in the chilly breeze. I stared indifferently as they played their game, but secretly envied them that death had not entered their lives this weekend.

I felt the heavy footsteps from within the building and turned back to the windows just in time to catch a close-up of the man dressed in black approaching the other side of the door. I lowered myself from tiptoe and quickly straightened my jacket one last time.

The lock jingled and the door opened.

"Good afternoon," the chubby man said.

I was the first to enter and shook the man's comfortable hand.

"I'm terribly sorry for your loss," he said.

"Thank you," I replied solemnly.

Having made it past him, I wasted no time in entering the viewing room. A small rectangular sign hung on the wall by the entrance. The white letters against the black background spelled out my grandmother's name: *Maria Alaimo.*

"Thank you, Mr. LoMorte." I heard my father say.

My busy eyes followed the rows and rows of chairs in the dark paneled room. Starting at the back of the room I worked my gaze toward the front to three crimson armchairs keeping watch over Nonna's casket.

I walked softly and alone to the front of the room and stood capturing every nuance. The smell of the flowers, the lights behind the casket that cast a warm glow over Nonna's features. And the light shroud covering my grandmother from her hands to her feet seemed to envelope her like a soft cloud.

"That's why she looked all misty from the window," I whispered to myself, standing to the side of the dark paneled walls. With my hands crossed behind me I whispered, "Hi, Nonna."

She looked as though she was sleeping and I was afraid to wake her. Her makeup was a bit caked on her face and lips. Her mouth protruded a bit. "Probably because of the stitches keeping her mouth closed," I thought morbidly.

I approached and knelt on the cushioned kneeler. Her hands clasped a rosary. The beadwork on the dress sparkled like diamonds. Josephine had made a good choice to bury her in this purple gown despite the fact that this was not reflective of the simple grandmother I knew on a daily basis. But it wouldn't have been appropriate to bury her in one of the sleeveless dresses made by her own hands.

Today she was dressed for a special occasion, and this would definitely qualify as a special occasion. The gown was long and covered the entirety of her legs. Her shoes were visible from beneath the layers of chiffon. I could clearly see that her right foot was somewhat bent to the inside. This was the leg that had announced the return of her cancer that cold January day nine months earlier.

Up until this point most of my thoughts concentrated on my surroundings, the external qualities of the day, and not once on my internal feelings—until I knelt by the coffin. While I accepted my inability to cry, I was greatly comforted to have her within sight and touch.

I rested my chin in my cupped hands gazing at the rosary that hung on the inside casket lid. Its small, budding roses entwined delicately with a silvery chain.

From the rosary hung the names of her grandchildren: Charles, Maria, Mark, and Annamaria, all emblazoned with gold lettering on the red satin ribbon.

My knees creaked as I rose from the kneeling position. I made the sign of the cross in front of the large wooden crucifix centered on the wall above the coffin and flanked on either side by dark crimson velvet curtains, each pulled back from center.

I took a seat in the fifth row of regular folding chairs. It was a while before anyone else arrived and gave me a chance to ponder where Nonna was now. I imagined her looking down, having made the journey to the other side. What did she feel? Could she see us? Was she now with all the saints to whom she prayed to each and every day?

My Aunt Josephine and Uncle Michael were the next visitors. My head tilted to the right as I watched Nonna's daughter stand beside the coffin and wipe tears from her eyes.

Michael decided to give her some time alone and joined me. I got up off my seat and extended my hand.

"Hey, Michael."

"Hi, Charlie," he said calmly.

We walked to the back of the room where a podium stood. A mourner sign-in book lay open on the tilted top. Michael signed for him and Josephine. I followed my uncle's lead and did the same. At the top ledge of the podium were small wooden pockets that held a multitude of saint cards commemorating Nonna's death. They witnessed each and every signature.

I grabbed a bunch of the two by three-inch laminated cards and went through them like a collector.

Saint Theresa, Saint Jude, Saint Anthony…

I quickly shuffled through the small stack. The choices were seemingly endless, but finally I made my selection—Our Lady of Fatima. I turned the card over to read the inscription. Although this one happened to be in Italian, I understood it quite well.

In amata memoria di
MARIA ALAIMO
Morta il 19 Settembre 1981
Interment St. Raymond's Cemetery
Section Pieta, Range…

I read the words back to myself in English. "In loving memory of Maria Alaimo, died on September 19, 1981."

The shuffle of more visitors broke the silence of the immediate family. Looking past the decorated wreaths and cascades of floral arrangements placed along the wall on thin green metallic stands, I was overcome by the perfume emanating from the fragrant blossoms.

At the front stood an arch made of white carnations and beneath it a podium covered with the same flowers. A book made of Styrofoam and lettered in black lay on the podium. It was inscribed "Maria Alaimo. Born September 28, 1920. Demise September 19, 1981."

"Demise?" I thought. What a hideous word, so cold and callous.

My *bisnonni*, or great-grandparents had entered the room.

Papa Diego came in holding onto Grandma Rosalia's arm. Clothed in a dark blue coat and kerchief, she wailed loudly. Her small, four foot nine inch frame barely cleared the brown-coppered casket bottom. Her eyes, barely visible through her wrinkled skin, gave the appearance that she was smiling, not crying.

"Maria!" my great-grandmother yelled in her raspy voice. "Maria!" she yelled once more before she threw herself at her stepdaughter's lifeless body. That's all that was needed to send everyone in the room into a fit of hysterics. Crying and wailing echoed off the walls in the room. I observed the scene from my seat.

Grandma Rosalia had let go of the casket and was now supported by Concettina, who brought a white handkerchief to her nose and eyes. Trailing behind the elderly couple were their other children Antonia and Sal.

Papa Diego was more subdued. He held onto the wooden kneeler and sobbed softly. "Maria," he said. He dabbed his eyes gazing at his firstborn. At ninety-three years of age, he probably never anticipated outliving one of his own children.

"Maria! Maria! Maria," my great-grandmother continued to wail.

"Oh my God," Uncle Michael muttered in disbelief at the whole scene.

The wake was now underway, the dramatics and placement could not have been any better had a Hollywood producer been directing the scene.

Those who weren't crying whispered to their neighbor without moving their heads. They put on a good show playing the parts of good Italian mourners in their black garments and even darker faces. They sat stoically never moving except for their thick, rough fingers that showed years of laborious work but they were dexterous and agile enough to never miss a bead on their rosary. Their eyes scanned the room looking who was present, and more importantly, how those present were behaving. All they cared about was how they were perceived—good mourners showing respect for the deceased.

Nonna hated attending wakes and often sent Nonno in her place. The one thing I understood very early on was the importance of showing up at 'these things' as my father sometimes referred to them.

Like many Italian families, my family never forgot those people who did not come to pay respects. If you didn't show up at one of your relative's wakes, they sure as hell were not going to show up when one of your family members passed away.

There were relatives in that twenty-five by seventy-five foot room that I hadn't seen in years. They were not distant relatives, but Aunts who sort of lost touch after Nonno fought with them; a fight that erupted four years earlier when I was hospitalized and almost died.

My grandfather had been working on the Long Island Expressway when a drunk driver hit him that fateful May evening in 1977. Dad had rushed to the hospital telling my family it was the worse accident he had ever witnessed. Nonno's intestines, all of his insides, were out and lying atop his body with blood everywhere.

I had visited Nonno a number of times. He was swathed in bandages from head to foot; two broken arms and both legs no better off. Yet, despite the odds he pulled through. One doctor commented that the only reason Nonno survived was due to his strong heart. "A heart like a horse," he had said.

When my grandfather emerged from his white cotton cocoon, all he could think about was how his two stepsisters were trying to get their hands on his land in Sicily. It was the same land I had the pleasure of visiting with him in August 1982 when we toured Italy and Sicily.

Had it not been for the four rocks in each corner of the parched barren parcel, I would have missed this patch of earth altogether. What a shame this piece of earth had brought so much mistrust among siblings.

Aunt Concettina held onto Papa Diego's arm and helped him to a seat in the second row. The same height as her father, it was a struggle for her to support him and make sure he didn't lose his balance.

I continued surveying the room for a while then stared straight ahead at the woman whose company and simplicity I had come to idolize over the past year. There were so many years that were wasted because of my youth and lack of realization of just how special she was. I again tried to imagine where she might be at this very moment. Was she standing in the corner looking out onto the now growing crowd?

I felt a tickle on my top lip and used my tongue to wipe the salty tear away. I hoped heaven was everything she expected. I sat relishing the thought of actually knowing someone on the other side now.

I crossed my arms and sunk deep into my seat secure in the knowledge that I now had someone to watch over me, someone who could tap St. Anthony or St. Jude on the shoulder and send them my way.

14

Goodbye, but not Forever

Tuesday morning greeted me with blue skies, a cool wind, stomach flips, and a distinct uneasiness. The feeling had been building over the past three days since I first heard the news Nonna had died.

The day I knew would inevitably come, was now here.

I was confused, upset and lost in the truest sense. Though only a mere teenager, my life had not been easy, and peace of mind for me was hard to come by. The past few days were now filled with inconsequential actions devoid of meaning. A radio blared in the background; an announcer yelling about cars. I sat emotionless at the dining table holding my clean-cut chin against the knuckles of my right hand and pondering the stupidity and sheer insignificance of the radio commercial.

"What difference does all this marketing and consumerism mean when in the end we all wind up dead," I thought.

I stared ahead oblivious to the news, songs, ads and things that could do nothing for me at that moment. They couldn't bring my grandmother back and only served to remind me of when she was alive. Like the song I had heard only two days before her death. Thinking of that song now only made me wish I could go back to the first time I heard it and change things somehow.

◆   ◆   ◆

We entered the funeral parlor one last time.

The priest having concluded the final blessing, invited all family and friends to come up to the casket to say their final goodbye.

The throngs came and went from the casket, starting with Nonna's sisters and brother-in-laws. Some hugged her and others kissed her forehead. The group whittled down to the immediate family and before I realized, it was my turn. All I could muster was to pat my grandmother gently on her forearm. It was hard.

The chiffon material on her arm moved back and forth against her skin. I felt myself beginning to cry. Uncontrollable sobs started. The three days of swelling that had been buried deep inside me were finally released as I removed my hand from the mesh-like shroud that covered her.

I was never going to see her again. Ever.

I stood by the doorway at the foot of her casket. My crying was now intense. I watched my father kiss Nonna's forehead. My heaves were forceful and my arms swayed as I tried to control the convulsions enveloping my body.

With everyone having said their final goodbyes, the funeral director's staff closed the coffin. I looked on, leaning my body against the frame of the doorway. The lid of the coffin slowly closed. Nonna's face disappeared beneath the lid. I caught one final glimpse of her purple gown and the bottom of a shoe. With a final light click, the casket was locked.

Nonna was instantly gone, sealed off from the rest of her family forever.

Josephine tried to comfort me to no avail. My face hurt from squinting. My eyes were red and swollen. Tears from my drenched cheeks dripped onto my black blazer. There was no comforting me.

During the short limo ride to Immaculate Conception Church, I felt no better. My family stood mingled in front of the light brick edifice. The sweet and cool September breeze comforted us as we watched Nonna's glossy coffin lifted out of the hearse and onto the shoulders of the pallbearers.

"You bigga boy, no crya," Aunt Antonia chided me. It only caused me to cry more.

We followed Nonna into the church. My sobbing had subsided, but the residual effect of my heaving could be heard throughout the vast open space and echoed from the arched walls and the statues of saints lining either side of the church. As I passed the brown-robed St. Anthony I was able to manage a slight genuflect. My vision blurry from tears caused Nonna's draped coffin to be a big blur. I wasn't able to regain focus.

"Family and friends, we are…" the priest began as I gazed upward toward the altar and the five-foot crucifix hanging there, the body of Christ and all my sorrows affixed to it. "…here to celebrate the life and death of Maria."

The sorrowful hymns during services brought a resurgence of my tears. Out of everyone present I was the most visibly upset by all this.

Loud sobs interspersed with the singing of hymns and readings echoed through the church.

In a short forty-five minutes the service came to an end.

The family followed Nonna as her casket was carried down the aisle. The recessional song, *Morning has Broken* was played on the church's organ. I thought it an odd selection and looked up to see a brown-haired woman belting out the tune. It was not the typical Catholic hymn, but it worked for me.

After interment ceremonies at St. Raymond's, Nonna's physical presence was officially no longer with us.

That comfortable late summer day ended with a feast of antipasti and cold cuts, sliced Italian bread and rolls, and of course, family and friends. I sat alone on the plastic covered gold sofa watching everyone eat in the room where I had shared so many dinners and Sunday coffee visits with my grandmother.

It had only been three days since her death, but life was already different. The house felt different. I knew my life was never going to be the same and sensed the enormity of these recent events. I felt lost as if I had wandered into a black hole, a dream from which I would awake to find out that the past three days had been made up. My empty gaze caught the attention of my father in the front dining room.

"Come and eat something." His voice broke my trance.

"No," I said softly, shaking my head.

With Nonna's death, so came the end of summer. Before I knew it I would too soon be thrust into the reality of everyday life.

◆   ◆   ◆

Toward the end of the week I was called to my grandmother's house once again, but this time to assist Josephine in going through Nonna's clothes for the purpose of donating them to charity.

I wanted to be there, not so much to help out my aunt, but to perhaps find and keep a memento of my grandmother. Her night table drawers were a virtual treasure chest of memorabilia. Although the day was a beautiful one, my walk to Nonna's was anything but. There was no urgency on my part. I took my time retracing the steps that Nonna had traveled many times.

I closed my eyes as I walked under the train overpass and pictured Nonna walking up the block as she had done so many times before. I put my memory to the test trying to see if the game had paid off. It didn't. I could not remember her to the level of detail that I had hoped.

Josephine went through the large wooden closet removing many of Nonna's dresses. They were all the same style, though some were sleeveless and some had cap sleeves. All were navy or brown and all handmade. Now they were going to a new home, perhaps to another Grandma.

I didn't want to get in the way of my aunt's tasks. These were her mother's items. I watched her while I sat on the edge of the bed dangling my long legs over the side. My hands along my side supported me and I was comforted by the softness of the cotton duvet. It was the same place Nonna had sat so many times.

I realized for the first time that my father had lost his mother, and a deeper sense of loss overtook me. With my left knee now curled up on the bed, I felt the warmth of the sun coming in through the slats of the open blinds. Every now and then a light breeze came through the open window. The sheer, beige panel curtains occasionally billowed, the movement graceful and serene. The sweet smelling breeze was soothing as I drew it up into my nostrils.

Finally the moment had come. Josephine went to the nightstand. The stout shiny wood dresser had two drawers filled with religious articles and items of a more personal nature. I reached for the ornate gold handle. My mind raced, thinking of the treasures behind the curved and beveled façade.

The top drawer contained her old eyeglasses, gray with a light beige trim encircling each lens, and stored in a gold embroidered case. Josephine threw them into the steel trashcan in the kitchen. I quickly salvaged them, but not before a bit of tomato sauce from within the trashcan soiled the ornately embroidered fabric case.

As I expected, there were also a myriad of prayer cards, many of Padre Pio.

"Here's a card with a wooden cross," I mumbled to myself. "Hmm. It says 'Made with wood from the Garden of Gethsemane." I could not discard this and instead made a small pile of things I would keep.

I came across one holy card depicting a man wearing a long black robe and surrounded by children. I knew who he was even before I turned the small laminated card over. It was St. John Bosco.

Two years earlier in June 1979, Nonna had bought me a beige, four-inch plastic statue of St. John after whom my middle name was given. This small statue became a cherished relic.

◆   ◆   ◆

Tony was sitting in the yard this warm June evening. From the far side of the kitchen through the open screen door, Charles heard the voices of his grandparents. He went to the door and looked out. His father was setting up two folding chairs for his parents. He quickly joined them and kisses were had all around.

His father stepped into the house for a moment to turn on the porch light, the only illumination for the backyard. It cast a warm glow onto the group underneath the metal awning, Nonna wore her signature kerchief, and she and the elder Charles sat on the red and white striped chairs. Charles and Tony, father and son, opted for the hard gray concrete stoop.

The visit was unexpected and that made it even more special for the young boy.

Charles made out from the conversation among the group of adults that his grandparents had just returned from Manhattan and the feast of St. Anthony in Little Italy. Nonna reached into her black handbag and pulled out a light brown paper bag folded neatly at the top. The small six-inch square bag crinkled in her fingers as she handed it to her grandson.

"Questa e per te." She told him the bag was for him.

Charles opened it and peeked in before pulling out the four-inch plastic statue of St. John Bosco, the body, monotone beige, sat atop a black intricately engraved base and his head was capped with a thin, gold, metal halo. Only he had received a gift that evening. The statue would adorn the top of his dresser for many years to come.

◆   ◆   ◆

That statue like everything Nonna touched became very important to me. Like an artist's work that increases in value only after death, everything that belonged to Nonna, items she had touched or were special to her in her life, like the statue she had given to me, were now priceless.

15

Nonna Visits Again

I did not mean anything malicious by the term, but what I would refer to years later as 'the most welcome distraction of my life,' was now over.

I was grateful to have cared for Nonna that summer. I felt it was fate that much of these events came at a time when I could care for her. Although my helping Nonna may have seemed one-sided, little did anyone know that Nonna also helped me a great deal—by providing perspective. She taught me that things were not as bad as I pictured. She drew me away from my own concerns and gave me the courage I would need later in life to tackle problems and issues yet to be faced.

◆   ◆   ◆

The greenery of the landscape changed to the soft and inviting warmth of autumn colors. The death I had experienced two weeks earlier had not stopped the world around me. My world, as much as I hated to admit, went forward. But life was different now.

The soft fog that had enveloped me for the last six weeks was beginning to burn off. The days that separated us grew, and as quickly as the days passed, things started to change. Everything seemed to fall into place as if my grandmother's death had been the catalyst; a catalyst for my reawakening, of having greater confidence in myself, of looking at life with a renewed sense of promise that I did not want to spend at the mercy of others or what they thought of me.

The weather during the last week of September was cool and sky blue. On my way home from school, I decided to fulfill Nonna's wish that I look for a job at La Guli Pastry Shop. I was finally doing what Nonna asked me to do so many times during those bedside chats that summer.

I got the job. What I didn't know at the time was that this was where I would meet my future wife.

For me, the hardest parts of those months following Nonna's death were the simplest of tasks, like getting up in the morning. I had become conditioned to getting up, getting ready, and getting out of the house to help her, and now nothing. I was going through withdrawal.

Most of the time I awoke thinking she was still alive. For a brief moment between sleep and reality, my mind gave in to my wishes and it seemed Nonna was still alive.

Then reality hit, the cruelest moment of all. But even so, I knew somehow she was still with me. After all, she had visited me the evening on the day she died. I didn't need any other proof. And at other times Nonna also made her presence known. This was especially true in the months leading up to my wedding in 1989.

◆   ◆   ◆

As was usual and customary, I was the second one in my family to go to bed each night. My father, without fail, was always the first. Our living space was on one floor and the bedrooms were within earshot of the television in the living room.

When I came home and found the house empty, I would immediately turn on the radio or TV so I'd have noise around me. I was afraid of silence. It always brought on my thoughts and fears about life, not fitting in, how I wished my life was, etc.

Two months before my November wedding I retired to my bedroom and closed the door. I had been feeling a sense of melancholy all day and this feeling was still with me as I slipped between the sheets and enjoyed the warm comforts of my bed. My legs were tight and tired. I was upset Nonna wasn't there to see me on this milestone event, the planning and preparation for my wedding. I tried to turn over and find a more comfortable position, but the tightly wrapped sheet prevented me from doing so. I yanked the sheet out a bit, thought of my grandmother, turned to face the wall and cried.

The tears tickled my nose as they dripped down my face. It was warm that night, and I had the bedspread pushed down to the foot of the bed. I stared at the beige wall, now black in the darkness.

I suddenly felt something. I was no longer alone.

Someone had sat on the edge of the bed directly behind me. I wasn't the only one in the tiny room that I shared with my brother, but I knew the door to my bedroom had been closed since I had gotten into bed.

My mind raced. I knew for sure that nobody had entered the room. I had not fallen asleep so couldn't be dreaming. In fact I was quite awake. Frozen by fear, I couldn't scream. I scanned the wall just a few inches from my face, and with skillful precision, I strategically placed the thin blue cotton sheet between my big toe and the one next to it, and carefully pushed the fabric from my body.

My eyes remained open and I continued to stare at the blank wall. I propped my body up with my right arm and slowly rose, never moving my gaze from the wall. My left foot made its way over the edge of the bed and down to the floor. I made a leap for the light switch.

For a brief moment I was afraid to turn around despite the light.

Gingerly, I turned my head. The light from the high fixture in the room made the shellac on the door appear wet. I shifted my gaze to the edge of the bed. I stared incredulously, not quite believing what I saw. There on the edge of the bed was an imprint in the sheet as if someone had been sitting there. The imprint was clearly discernable. The rest of the sheet was smooth but for the semicircular indention created just moments before.

After getting over the initial shock and realizing my stupidity, I became angry with myself. There was no reason for me to be scared. I knew who had been sitting there.

Nonna.

"Would I have seen her if I had just been brave enough to have turned around?" I questioned myself.

Nonna also made herself known in other ways—through dreams. In the weeks leading to our marriage, Lisa and I each had extraordinarily similar dreams involving Nonna.

◆   ◆   ◆

Charles strode along the sidewalk to Nonna's house. He recognized familiar marks in the concrete that had not changed since he was small. His strides were brisk and long. He was a man now. No longer the shy introverted kid.

The sun was out and felt warm. The breeze cooled him. He was happy to be visiting his grandmother. It had been too long. He climbed the stairs. His long legs took them two at a time and before he knew it he was at the landing. This time, however, he did not ring the bell and wait for Nonna to answer. She was expecting him. He knew this when he saw her through the glass storm door. She was sitting alone wearing a blue sleeveless dress and sipping a cup of coffee.

She looked up as her tall grandson came toward her along the linoleum-lined hall.
From her vantage point she had a direct view of the front entranceway, the light
drenching Charles from behind. She looked down to place the white porcelain cup
into the matching saucer. The cup hitting the saucer made a dainty click.

It was as if time had not passed. Nonna looked the same. Time had not touched
her. They had sat at this kitchen table so many times to lunch or have a quiet snack.

"Nonna, I'm getting married," Charles announced to his grandmother.

"I knowwa," she said, her broken English just as he remembered. He missed hear-
ing her voice. "I'mma very happy for you and a Lisa."

Nonna smiled. The dream was over.

◆   ◆   ◆

In my dream I was the one visiting Nonna, but in Lisa's dream, Nonna visited
her.

Lisa had the dream first, and a few days later I had mine.

She recounted for me how she was home alone in her dream. She heard a
knock at the door of their apartment. (We were really fortunate to have found a
great apartment with all the space we wanted in a two family walk-up. Sal and
Margie, the elderly couple who owned the brick house were our surrogate grandparents. We both felt extraordinarily lucky and blessed to have had the fortune to
have found one another.)

Lisa opened the door realizing the woman standing in front of her wearing a
simple dress was none other than my grandmother. Lisa was startled.

"I told her to come in and sit," Lisa told me. "But she refused saying she only
wanted to meet me."

"Wait," Lisa told my grandmother. "You can't go, Charlie would love to see
you."

"No," Nonna responded. "I needa to go."

◆   ◆   ◆

One Sunday after we had been married a few years, we were cleaning, trying
to get rid of a few things we had collected in our spacious two-bedroom apartment. I was in the small bedroom we used as a guest room. The room was bright
and the hardwood floors were a nice touch. The rest of the apartment was carpeted.

I grabbed a stack of papers and old clothes for the trashcan in the kitchen. As I walked into the gray-carpeted living room, which adjoined the kitchen and dining area, something caught my attention. A movement. The white top of the trashcan was spinning as if someone had hit it hard throwing in garbage! I knew Lisa hadn't been into the room recently. I stared at the domed plastic lid and watched it spin two more times before coming to a halt.

"Lee!" I called.

Lisa came running when she heard me. She was as amazed as me.

◆   ◆   ◆

Three years later in 1992, Lisa visited Marie, a psychic. This was the same woman Lisa had visited two years earlier, the one who was remarkably on target about everyone in the family. For this particular visit, Lisa had gathered pictures of various family and friends. She also brought a cassette recorder since the psychic allowed the sessions to be taped. There was a clear-cut purpose for Lisa's visit—her health.

Lisa had been battling crippling back pain for eight months. None of the doctors we had visited—including many Park Avenue specialists—could diagnose the problem. Lisa had been through every imaginable test, CAT scans and MRIs. The pain had gotten so bad at the beginning of the year that one doctor placed her on Valium and told her to lie on a flat surface.

Nineteen ninety-two did not start out well at all.

New Year's Day found Lisa drugged out and laying on a hard board on the gray-carpeted living room of our apartment. Her blonde hair sprawled around her head. All that was needed, I thought, was a chalk outline to complete the 'dead' look. She had slept on the floor the entire night. She could barely even talk because of the Valium.

I went down the three flights of stairs, hopped into our gray sedan and drove the short distance from our apartment on tree-lined Forty-second Street, to my parent's house.

"Why don't you stay?" my dad had asked, as I loaded veal cutlets, green beans, and pasta into a variety of Corning Ware. The smells were wonderful. I wanted to stay and eat over, but I was so exhausted and frustrated at everything that was going on, I just lost it and cried as I held the large bowl of lightly-battered veal chops.

"Charlie stop crying," Dad told me.

◆   ◆   ◆

Soon after her return from the psychic, Lisa phoned me at the office to tell me the results. I had waited a good part of the day to hear from her.

"So, what did she say?" I asked, as I sat at my desk and shuffled papers in no particular order. The blue striped tie around my neck seemed to strangle me.

"You're not going to believe it. She said we are going to have two children." (Besides Gabriella who was born in 1996, we would have a son Anthony in 2001.)

"No, I meant what did she have to say about what you're going through?"

"She asked if I had been tested for Lyme disease. She thinks this may be the reason." Her voice became a bit fuzzy through the static coming across the line. "And just wait till you hear what she had to say about you. She said tha—"

I stopped my wife midway. "Don't tell me until I get home."

We arrived home later that evening and I could not wait to hear the tape. I had been thinking about it all day and the anticipation had been building. I grabbed the black recorder just as Lisa inserted the tape. It clicked as it locked into position. Lisa's fingers hit the smooth black levers searching for the discussion relating to me.

She stopped the fast forward function and pressed play. "Do you see me—"

"That's not it," Lisa said, and stopped the tape mid-sentence. She once again hit the lever to advance the tape.

"He comes from sturdy stock. You'll need a shotgun to get rid of him." Lisa's laughter could be heard on the tape. I looked at her quizzically.

"She was referring to you."

"Oh!" I was pleasantly surprised. "That's great. I'm going to live a long life?"

There was some truth to the psychic's statements about coming from sturdy stock. All I had to do was look at Nonno and what he went through, not to mention a history of longevity in my family. My great-grandfather Papa Diego had lived to be ninety-nine years old.

"It should be coming up," Lisa said, as the tape continued in fast forward.

"My husband, he wants to know about…if there are any spirits ever with him," Lisa asked Marie. I could hear the shuffling of cards in the background.

There wasn't even a moment's hesitation before she responded quickly and unequivocally. "Yes. There's an older woman around him."

"Is there?" Lisa asked, amazement in her voice.

"Yeah. I don't get a mother; it's more like a grandmother."

"Yep, that's exactly who she is." Lisa sounded excited on the tape, but I didn't want her to give too much information to the psychic.

"And I get her as being very warm, and guiding him whenever possible," Marie advised Lisa. I thought this point was rather obvious. Aren't all grandmothers warm and guiding?

The tape continued after a brief silence. "And there are times when she either whispers in his ear or gives him signs that she's there. So he has to know."

I sat on the gray-carpeted floor amazed by what I heard. Now, I would never run and tell anyone in my family this because I always thought it was against Catholicism to visit psychics, mystics, or fortunetellers.

One week later, the psychic's predictions were somewhat validated. I had accompanied Lisa to NYU Medical Center for her next battery of tests. As we exited the hospital doors into the midmorning light, I headed for one cab and Lisa headed for another. I opened the door to mine and was struck by what I saw. Scattered across the floor of the yellow car were bills. Ones, fives, and few twenties.

I called over to Lisa motioning hard with my right hand for her to join me. "Lee, let's take this cab."

The psychic had seen Lisa coming into money and told her to play Lotto.

I slid across the blue vinyl seat and motioned for my wife to be calm, and then I pointed to the floor. Bills were scattered all about our feet. We discreetly picked the bills off the floor while carrying on a rather mundane discussion with each other.

At one point Lisa started chuckling at our unbelievable luck and nonchalantly bent down to grab a wad. When the bills were collected and counted our yield was $346!

Was it a coincidence that this occurred only a few days after Lisa's visit to the fortuneteller? I didn't know what to think. It was nice that this had happened and I was glad I had gone to a different cab. For me it validated what was revealed on the tape was true. I knew firsthand that Nonna was always with me, especially after my bout with anxiety disorder and all the visits she had paid me. I didn't need to confirm to anyone this truth.

Nonna would often visit at times of illness or crisis. One such visit was in 1990 when I began to suffer crippling bouts of anxiety.

◆   ◆   ◆

There's good reason when flying to keep your seatbelts fastened. Although the flight may be smooth and uneventful one minute, turbulence can come in and rob that feeling of security faster than you can latch the buckle or close the window shade.

The year was 1990. The year that would send Charles heading on a course of turbulence so severe he would need all the strength he could muster to fly out of it.

The storm clouds were forming in January as he began his journey into the new year. The dark gray and black cumulus billows reached for the upper echelons of the atmosphere blocking out the sun. Before he knew it, he was at the mercy of a turbulent storm; riding each updraft like a surfer on a fifty-foot wave and shuddering violently as he hit each air pocket.

In a few short months so much had changed in his life. The major event was his marriage in November of 1989. Lisa often cried over leaving her home and missing her family. Charles would laugh and told her to stop crying. He had looked forward to getting out of his house and starting his own life and found her rationale amusing. Until they returned from their honeymoon, and in a span of two weeks his outlook and life had changed.

Work wasn't the same. He was depressed upon returning from his office after his honeymoon to find his group had moved to a new section of the office. Even the walk home from the train station was different and torturous for him. As much as he needed change, Charles was also a creature of habit and familiarity. All the things he held in such contempt were the same things that grounded and defined him.

Lisa was the first to rescue him from the past. After Nonna's death the years rolled by quickly, each blurring into the next. There were moments when Charles was completely stuck, unable to move forward with his life. Although according to the calendar the years were surely changing—he wasn't.

Charles met Lisa innocently enough while working at the pastry shop where his aunt Josephine had worked many years prior, and where Nonna had urged him to visit and apply for employment. It was a bit ironic that only one year after her death Charles had applied and actually gotten a job there. He knew his grandmother had a hand in this.

One afternoon Charles was cleaning out the stainless steel cylinder ice machine. During the summer months it churned out crushed ice of every imaginable flavor including orange, strawberry, and Spumoni—the favorite of many customers. Charles' personal favorite was chocolate, which he often combined with the tangy and zesty lemon.

He stood atop the mosaic floor with a shiny steel bucket filled with hot, boiling water and proceeded to dump it into the hatch at the top of the machine. Above the din of the liquid hitting the spinning interior blades, a girl came into the room from the front of the store on her way to the freezers in the back. She wore a red smock, the standard uniform of La Guli girls. Her hair was blonde and pulled back from her face in a ponytail. Charles hadn't met her before. She came up to him with a dazzling smile and dazzling blue eyes to match. Her quick wave was comical as she approached him.

"Hi, my name's Lisa."

"Hi, ummm Charlie."

He had smiled slightly. Little did either one of them know this brief introduction was the beginning of their path through life together. It was all so mysterious and bigger than the both of them.

Isolation can come in many forms. For Charles, isolation had become a way of life. An art form perfected. He was accustomed to internalizing much of what he felt and experienced. Growing up with very few, if any true friends bothered him a great deal. As a teenager, it was awkward for him to introduce himself or even strike up a conversation, all the things that seemed to come easy for other people.

Charles' lack of self-confidence did not improve the situation. Not having friends was one thing, not having family he could talk to made his life even more difficult. How much of this was self-imposed nobody knew. Perhaps this behavior was a defense mechanism.

During the early years and indeed through life, Charles found his strength in the saints to whom he prayed each and every morning. They were entrusted with seeing him through the day to show him the way, and most of all to not give him more than he could handle. Sometimes they came through and sometimes not.

After his grandmother died, his faith in the saints was shaken. Nonna had trusted them to see her through her illness and they let her down. And they had let him down, too. Now there was the isolation once again as he battled these anxiety attacks. After visiting eight physicians, most told him he was fine. His last appointment, a cardiologist, diagnosed his affliction as severe anxiety disorder. The fact that the discomfort he was experiencing had a name was half the battle in overcoming an affliction that seriously curtailed his life. The other half of the cure, as Charles was to find out, would be his grandmother.

The attacks, which started with thoughts of death, began about the same time he had his tonsils removed in June of 1989. It was the first time he ever had surgery. Although the first three weeks following the operation were perhaps the most painful in his life, he managed. Every swallow was as if ten sharp steak knives were piercing the lining of his throat. Still, this discomfort was better than the delirious fevers he had suffered a week before the surgery from yet another bout (one of at least five per year) of tonsillitis.

Lisa had given him an ultimatum; get the tonsils out or they were not getting married. It was a joke of course, but her declaration was for Charles' benefit. Though soon after the surgery he started to feel, for lack of a better word, 'off.'

At first there were the occasional bouts of nausea, a bit of lightheadedness, always accompanied by a general feeling of doom. Initially, Charles discounted this as just nerves at the thought of his getting married in a few months. But the mild nausea and feeling of weariness soon reached a higher level of severity.

The middle of the night was the worse. He frequently awoke to a racing heart, profuse sweating, and the feeling he was not going to make it through the night alive. Sleep became a fearful activity. He was so afraid of dying while sleeping, the thought became an obsession. Sleep deprivation was a natural result and only served to fuel his tortuous thoughts of death.

During the day Charles was so tired and vulnerable that anxiety episodes would creep up on him unannounced and totally debilitate him. Even the simplest tasks became arduous. He could not walk to the store by himself or drive alone. "What if I died and I was alone?" was the one thought that ran through his head.

Some days he couldn't even ride the train, let alone go under the tunnel. On the days when he was able to make it into work, he had to talk himself through the attacks. By the time the train made it across Manhattan, he was so spent, the only choice for him was to get off at Lexington Avenue, cross the platform and ride the train home. He missed a lot of work during this time, and even while at work, the limitations placed on him by the anxiety rendered him unable to walk from his office, and down the hallway to the cafeteria.

By the time he and Lisa returned home from a long day of work, the constant thought of doom combined with the physical manifestations, exacted a harsh toll. It became a daily ritual for him to enter their apartment, head to the bedroom and cry.

Even the one thing he loved most, flying, was affected. One weekend after boarding a flight for Boston with Lisa and his sister, the feelings overtook him and he got off the 727 and went back to the gate.

By that summer the attacks peaked—seven or eight each day. His life had been full of change the past couple of months, from completing college, marriage, new apartment, and a new job. Even walking to and from the train station was an emotional ordeal. As his infliction grew, he felt himself drawn to his faith. He had felt himself growing apart from his religion. He wasn't attending Mass frequently and that was *beginning to bother him. His suffering was beginning to take on a spiritual dimension.*

During his battle he was drawn to the green rosary that had belonged to Nonna. Suddenly, and without explanation or sense, he began to recite the rosary each evening. To supplement this he read practically every book on the market about the apparitions of the Virgin Mother. From Fatima to Knock in Ireland, he could not get enough of the books or the information. He felt inexplicably drawn to the Blessed Virgin and to the rosary.

Even after the diagnosis he was still afflicted by anxiety, which periodically caught him off guard. Once he knew he was suffering from acute anxiety disorder, it was a tremendous relief to him. It was mental rather than physical. The fact that there was nothing wrong with his heart was a burden off his shoulders. Although knowledge is power, whenever he felt tired or rundown, the anxiety attacks began—a twinge in his stomach and a fluttering of his heart took over.

Charles often felt 'assured' by the people who helped him through this period of his life—the saints, the Virgin Mary, his grandmother. When he did experience an attack, infrequent though they may have been, he always felt as if he had let that group down. Charles experienced an example of this in a very vivid dream one evening after his racing heart and sweaty brow signaled the end of one such occurrence.

◆　　　◆　　　◆

He walked down a long stone corridor through pointed and regal Gothic arches that lined the one-hundred foot long hall. On the cobblestone walls in iron holders, candles danced lighting the way and playing off the walls.

As he entered a room off to the right of the corridor, an abundance of candles greeted him. Before him to his right stood a man, his torso protected by armor; a spear in his left hand.

"Why do ye still doubt after all you have been through?" Charles experienced no fear even though the stranger was visibly angered with him. Charles could not respond. He looked down at the stone floor and realized that though he was barefoot, he was not the least bit cold in this stone castle. He was more ashamed than anything at that moment.

"Do not fear anymore," the stranger in regal garb said, and the dream ended.

The next morning looking to satisfy his curiosity as to who the figure in his dream was, Charles looked at pictures of saints in the multitude of books and holy cards on his night table. He wanted to see if there might be any resemblance to the irate visitor he had seen in his dream. He sat on his bed in his shorts flipping through the books he had amassed over the years and finally came across a picture of St. Michael.

It was him! St. Michael had visited him. He had come to help Charles fight his battle.

Amazingly, once Charles told his family what he suffered from the stories began to come out. His father told him that his grandmother had suffered from the same thing. She was claustrophobic and could not even go to church because she would start having anxiety attacks.

"Come to think of it," Charles thought, "I never did see her attend a Sunday Mass. Instead, she always opted for just dropping in after a weekday Mass to light a candle."

◆   ◆   ◆

For me, the similarities of my illness and what Nonna had experienced was yet another sign that she was still with me, helping me to learn a lesson. However, it wasn't until after I had experienced this hard period in my life that I found out my grandmother had also suffered from anxiety as well.

16

Nineteen Years and Full Circle

The smell of the cleaning wax was everywhere in the room. It hung heavy in the early August air infiltrating the skylights of the family room. The dampness did not allow the lemony-mist to get very far above my head. With the effort of a man on a mission, I scrubbed the top of the oak coffee table with my left hand over my right until it shined. My strong back and forth motion had moved the square table out of place and I repositioned it ensuring it was still parallel to the green-checkered highboy. I grew increasingly anxious. I looked down at the green carpet to make sure the legs aligned with the already existing indentations. There was something gnawing at me, telling me that I needed to be elsewhere. But it was one of those rainy, damp and humid August Saturday afternoons and my energy level was way past low.

Anxiety is a strange thing. It can make a mockery of the sanest individual. Dealing with it can even be arduous. Some people eat out of nervousness, heading to the fridge to pull out the most decadent desert or treat. For me, however, I did not succumb to such delightful treats, but found solace and reparation by going to the broom closet to get a broom to start sweeping or a rag to dust the heck out of the house.

The only explanation that rationalizes this compulsion is that it came into being around the time I was helping Nonna clean her house. Cleaning was the one thing I could do to make her happy. The more I cleaned, the more I felt that in some way it would help her get better. She loved a clean house and for everything to be in order, and I was able to do these chores for her.

Lisa emerged at the top of the family room stairs and looked down. I was fidgety, unable to focus on the television. I looked up.

"I feel like I need to be there right now," I told her, my voice aggravated.

"So go. What do you want me to say?" she said, with a hint of anger in her voice. I hated when she spoke to me like that. I was damned if I did and damned if I didn't. Or maybe it was just the anger within me for sitting there. I wanted to relax, but I knew I should be at the hospital. It was the kind of inner struggle that consumed me all the time. The simplest of decisions were always long and drawn out. What I knew to be right deep inside often clashed with what I *really* wanted to do. During these constant battles I always grew frustrated and angry with myself, and with whoever happened to be around me at that time.

By the time I left the house, it had been nearly three hours since I received the phone call from my mother who told me things were not looking good for Nonno. Now it was five o'clock and the afternoon was fading.

The red door thumped closed behind me. I headed down the slate steps to the car. As I fumbled for my keys, a light breeze scattered water from the leaves of a tree. The drops fell on my head flattening my graying hair and soaking through the shoulders of my blue t-shirt.

Almost forty minutes later, after getting caught in traffic generated by a ball game at Shea, I arrived at the hospital. I was lucky enough to find parking right up the block from the hospital. I got out and strode toward the all too familiar building.

I got off the elevator at the fourth floor and was happy to finally be out of that stinking slow lift. Sneakers squealing against the tiled floor, I made a quick left turn at the nurse's station. My rapid gate almost caused me to bump into Uncle Michael. He was escorting Martha, Nonno's wife, home. I raised my hand and gave a faint hello not missing a step as I walked right by them.

Lisa had visited Nonno two days earlier. Prior to heading to Nonno's room that day, she purchased one single red rose for him. That's all she could buy with the money she had with her. When she arrived at Nonno's room, Martha asked Lisa who the rose was for.

Thinking it a stupid question, Lisa replied, "It's for you, Martha."

I was furious when I heard the story. "Who the hell was in the hospital bed? It should have been obvious who the rose was for!"

No sooner had my grandfather and Martha met in a senior citizen club, only a few years after Nonna passed away, she had her hooks in him. They were married with a full-blown ceremony at Immaculate. There was no shame.

What hurt me the most was how Nonno did things with her that he never did with Nonna. He traveled one year to the Dominican Republic, Martha's native land, then they took a cruise the following year.

I harbored a great deal of resentment, much of which I tried to dismiss and refuse to recognize, but it was still there. The bitter feelings every now and then swelled within me, and at times I did not know where to direct them. Most of the time my feelings were toward my grandfather for marrying this woman, and then doing things with her he never did with Nonna, such as the traveling and gift buying.

As for Martha, I thought she was no more than a gold digger hidden behind tight gaudy dresses, designer frames and a white wig. She was everything my grandmother was not—classless, egotistical, and materialistic. She was so unlike my grandmother who made her own dresses (whether from her love of sewing or the fact my grandfather was cheap—I never quite knew). Nonno's second wife looked through every magazine possible for ideas of what to purchase next, and when it came to preparing meals, forget it. Her cooking was so bad at one point Nonno thought she was trying to kill him. Similarly, Martha always threw accusations at her in-laws, insinuating *they* were trying to kill *her*.

"No, no I get sick fromma the coffee, jes at Josephine's." She once accused my aunt of trying to poison her when she allegedly got sick from a cup of coffee. This behavior made my dad very nervous. Whenever Martha was invited to family barbeques or the like, he always treated Martha with kid gloves—yet another thing I hated about this union.

When it came to a party and food it was miraculous how Martha would lose her cane and run to the buffet tables. For me, watching her plump figure with her gray-coiffed hair run lickety-split to the food was more entertaining than the music. Her agility was remarkable if a free buffet was before her. And it was not like she went only once. No. It was always two or three trips to gorge, ensuring her figure remained forever stocky beneath her tightly wrapped chiffon gowns and fake mink stoles.

Worse of all, my grandfather allowed himself to be sucked into all this. Although by the time he realized his error, it was too late and the family was left holding the ball and trying to figure out what to do.

I took great pleasure in the fact she was leaving the hospital that evening, and perhaps leaving our lives for good. I detested how uncomfortable her presence made everyone feel because we needed to be careful of what we said or did.

I slowed my pace as I entered Nonno's room. From ten feet away I could make out the black-garbed figure of my aunt standing by my grandfather's bedside. My wet and squeaky sneakers announced my presence. All acknowledged me as I entered the crowded room. All except my grandfather.

Nonno was already in very good company. Besides my dad, also present were Aunt Josephine and Diego, Aunt Olivia, Aunt Antonia and Maria Pia, and Aunt Maria and Uncle Sal.

"Hi, Nonno," I said forcefully.

Josephine's dark hair swayed back and forth around her white face as she leaned over the railing to pat her father's arm. "Papa, Charlie e qui." (*Dad, Charlie is here.*)

He opened his eyes briefly, but it was enough time for me to smile at him. Aunt Antonia sitting in the chair, fumbled through her black shiny borsa, her eyes and fingers scanning each corner of the pocketbook. They emerged successful—a clear plastic bottle with a blue cap held victoriously by her thumb and forefinger. Upon closer inspection I saw the bottle was in the shape of the Virgin Mary. Unscrewing the top Antonia sprinkled the wet contents all over her immobilized brother-in-law.

I just looked at her as she went about dabbing the liquid onto my grandfather's legs. I wanted to ask her what she was doing, but didn't. I knew she meant well. After all, she had been married to Nonno's brother Angelo, who had died from cancer in 1995. Nonno was the only link that held the two families together. My grandfather was never the same after his brother—his constant walking companion to and from Steinway to buy meat or just to walk—had died.

As I looked up and smirked at Josephine, Aunt Antonia lifted up the white sheet that was neatly tucked in at Nonno's feet exposing his legs. She spoke Italian to Olivia, the both of them feeling my grandfather's legs. From the way their hands prodded and patted, his legs had grown hard and cold, practically petrified I thought. His ashen skin barely provided enough cover for his bones.

"Toucha," Aunt Antonia prodded me.

"No thanks," I replied, and shook my head. There was no need for me to participate. I didn't need the tactile reality to confirm what my eyes already knew.

"The doctor asked us if we had made the arrangements." My father was speaking quietly to Maria Pia. His right hand held up his unshaved chin. "So, Diego and I went to Farenga."

"Farenga." I said.

Farenga's was a local funeral parlor on Ditmars Boulevard. I looked at Diego who had accompanied Dad. "Wow, the doctor really told you to make arrangements?"

"Yeah," he said quietly, his bushy mustache hid his upper lip. My uncle was younger than my dad, but at that moment he looked just as old. Knowing my father, this pronouncement must have been a harsh reality for him.

"How did my father take it?" I asked my uncle. Since I knew my dad all too well and how he would always convince himself that things were better than what they really were, having a doctor ask you if you made 'arrangements' must have been shocking.

I halfheartedly chuckled to myself thinking if I weren't here at the hospital my father would have told me that everything was fine. "Yeah Charlie, Nonno looks good," was the constant response I received from him.

Over the past four days, despite the fact that he tried to hide it, I realized just how much my father had aged. His hair was grayer and his mood more reserved, even when my daughter Gabriella came by to visit.

Dad was not demonstrative with his emotions. Talking about illness, whether his or someone else's, was awkward for him at best. I was concerned he was keeping too much bottled up inside with little or no discussion about Nonno's rapidly deteriorating health. Like a soda can that had just been shaken, I was worried my dad was bound to explode. As I watched his pensive gaze I couldn't help but imagine what he was thinking. Perhaps the same thing as his son. That with Nonno's death, logically, he would be next and then of course, ultimately that would lead to my own demise. I wasn't ashamed to think it. It was reality. In some way, as we all watched Nonno die, we were all dying.

The hours passed slowly in that confined hospital room. Each of us trying to take our minds off of what was inevitably going to occur that evening. Like the rain that cascaded down the window, the anecdotes began to flow.

"Do you remember when Uncle Charlie took out the whole row of car mirrors down on Thirty-sixth Street?" Maria Pia said.

We all laughed about the time when my grandfather lost his sense of proximity and drove his blue car into a row of parked cars taking out every side mirror. At the time it wasn't funny since someone could have been seriously injured. My dad had pleaded with his father to stop driving, but the senior Charles was not about to listen to anyone's suggestions. He was too stubborn.

Our laughter was pleasantly interrupted by some familiar faces, those of my young cousins, Angela and Rosalia. Their father, my uncle Vinny, was going home tonight after being hospitalized for close to two weeks. With one lung left and emphysema brought on by years of smoking, his going home was good news. But my cousins did not forget to visit their uncle Charles now lying before them.

The girls' faces, like craggy seaside bluffs, showed signs of weathering many storms as a result of their dad's illness. Angela was crying as she left the room. Having kissed her uncle goodbye, she knew it would be the last time.

◆   ◆   ◆

Angela and Rosalia were spared further grief for another month. Then suddenly on the morning of September fifteenth, Uncle Vinny collapsed while getting out of bed.

Unable to be revived, he died in his son Jack's arms. Of course, Charles was in San Francisco when he received the news.

"Your mom called," Lisa told him when he phoned to advise his 767 had touched down safely.

"Oh, so who died?" he joked, not knowing of the death of Uncle Vinny.

"Uncle Vinny," she replied.

The smile disappeared from his face. He wasn't expecting news like this, he thought as he rode in a cab to the hotel. Once again his parents who had found out much earlier that day, had decided not to call their son directly to tell him of the death in the family, rather they chose to wait and tell Lisa.

Charles was beginning to feel frightened of being away on a business trip. It seemed that every time he went away someone got ill or just plain ol' died. Luckily though, he would have time to say goodbye at his uncle's wake next Sunday afternoon, two hours after his plane arrived back at JFK.

◆　　　◆　　　◆

We stood by Nonno's bedside watching, waiting, and wondering when he would stop breathing. Aunt Antonia gave him an occasional once over to check the status of things. Every now and then she would dip a paper towel in a small cup of water and place it to his crusted lips.

Nonno lurched forward with each deep, slow breath. He was putting up a good fight. At one point it seemed like he wanted to say something. His jaw moved, the form of the bones visible beneath his skin.

"Che, Papa?" (*What, Dad?*) Josephine tried to encourage him to get the words out, but to no avail.

In the dim light we all held our breath and watched Nonno fight to hang on. My dad, his right hand still supporting his chin, stood behind my younger cousin Maria. Diego and Olivia remained at the foot of the bed. On the right side of Nonno were Antonia, Josephine and me. Aunt Mariutsa and Uncle Sal stood near the doorway.

There was a shuffle at the door and Aunt Mariutsa stepped aside to let a nurse through.

"Excuse me, but we are here to change the sheets," she politely told the group. "We just need to ask you to step into the hallway."

I left the room and glanced down the nondescript hallway to the large round clock hung on the far wall. Its black hands read eight forty. I leaned against the smooth mauve wall, a few feet away from the rest of my family. My backside rested on my hands.

I was upset and confused. After all Nonno had been through this was how it was going to end. He had his family around him, which was more than could be said for a lot of people. But for me the lingering question was what to make of all this? I studied the faces of my family standing in the hall. My right foot was now flat against the wall, but not so far up as to draw attention or a reprimand from the staff.

"Look at all of us," I thought quietly. "Nonno is very lucky indeed."

Not only was my grandfather lucky, but so was my dad. Seeing the comfort he took in having his brother and sister with him made me realize the synergies between them. Diego had a much tougher skin than Dad and was already staking out a plan about what to do with Martha. Manipulation was not one of my dad's strong suits. He was so much like his mother in that respect. She always thought of the good in people. This was one time where I agreed there had been enough good. Josephine was much more like Diego and the three built on one another's strengths.

"I feel like we're just waiting for something to happen. No, Josephine?" My dad looked at his younger sister. She wore black pants, her feet crossed at the ankles. Her arms never moved from their crossed position over her chest and blue-flowered scarf. She indicated 'no' by moving her head back and forth, her lips curling upward to the right, her eyes never looking in my direction.

"It's nice that she's not here," she responded curtly. "Daddy's probably enjoying our company and conversation too much to go. He would have been gone already if she was here."

Josephine's words made me laugh out loud. The sheer sarcasm was way too enjoyable. I knew who she was referring to.

Up until recently Lisa and I had been talking quite a bit as to whether or not to have another child. I was concerned with Gabriella growing up an only child. I did not want her to go through what was playing out in this hospital room by herself. I did not want her to be alone when my and Lisa's time came. I did not want her to be the only one to pick out the casket and pick up the pieces and grieve alone. This was so very important to me. I did not want my now three-year-old daughter to be alone in life without the support of a brother or sister. While my own relationship with my siblings was somewhat stressed at times, I valued knowing they were there.

The fabric partition in the room rustled pulling my gaze away from the group. I pushed myself off the wall and peered through the door. With my arms crossed,

I leaned my head to the right just in time to see the nurse emerge from behind the curtain carrying soiled linens.

"It's okay, you can go in," she said, never looking back at us as she walked to the receptacle ten feet away to dump her haul.

The others lingered in the hallway not rushing back into the room. I took the opportunity to go inside and spend a quiet moment alone with Nonno. I walked to the far side of the bed and touched wisps of my grandfather's gray hair that had fallen over his forehead. He was in a different position now, his head facing the ceiling. I could tell this was a much more difficult position for my grandfather to be in to breathe.

"Don't worry, Nonno," I heard myself say as I touched his arm. I couldn't believe that a life was coming to an end. My grandfather had seen so much, done so much, and now here he was lying somewhere between here and there, wherever there was.

While my faith was strong at times, it was natural for me to question. I knew that before the night was over, I would know another person on the other side. His gasps came in thirty-second waves. He gulped air like a fish out of water. His chest heaved forward with every gasp. Gasp. Exhale. Gasp. Exhale. Finally and without warning, no more breaths. He had stopped breathing.

"Oh God, I can't be in here alone," I frantically thought to myself and ran out into the hallway.

"Hey guys, he stopped breathing!"

The group quickly regrouped and took their former places around the bed. I lagged behind waiting for them to assemble. Josephine lowered her left arm to touch her father's. "God will take care of you," she cried.

I slowly entered the room again and sat on the wood arm of the big leather chair. My leg went numb as the flat arm pressed against my sciatic nerve. I cried as I watched my aunt and father, who were hunched over the bed touching the white blanket covering Nonno's legs.

There were no more breaths. Nonno's bony face just stared ahead. The only sign of life was his barely moving Adam's apple. He was still fighting, still being Nonno, refusing to give in. His shocking pale blue eyes appeared serene. Gone was the fearfulness they had conveyed just an hour before. He seemed ready to go on this great journey. What did his eyes see before him? I wished at that moment to have a glimpse of what he was ready to embark on. Were there people ready to greet him? Was Nonna there?

Nonno had passed quietly at eight fifty with his closest family surrounding him and wishing him well. Like all those times I accompanied my dad to see him off at the airport on his flights to Italy, we were once again wishing Nonno *buon viaggio*; while his family and friends on the other side were wishing him *benvenuti*.

"He died!" Maria Pia's sudden and loud wail pierced the silence. She began crying hysterically.

The suddenness and intensity of her outburst shocked the others.

"Okay Maria," Josephine comforted her cousin. She placed her arm around the sobbing woman. "Okay." Her left hand squeezed Maria's arm above her elbow in an attempt to keep her sobs down for the sake of the other two patients in the room.

"But, but..." she could hardly speak. "He died on my birthday."

August twelfth was a date that would now have a double meaning in the family's calendar; beyond the happiness of a birthday, it was now the anniversary of a passing.

"You see," Josephine spoke in a calm and hushed voice still holding Maria's arm. "He gave you something to always remember him by. When it's your birthday, you will always remember this. He cared about you so much."

"And...an..." Maria stuttered on her first word as the sobs shook her body. "I loved him." She punctuated the sentence with another loud wail.

This was the first time I had ever seen someone pass away. I was amazed. I had been present at a birth but never a death. I had witnessed something incredible. The end of a life on earth.

Nonno made dying look easy. It was effortless the way my grandfather just stopped breathing. There was no thrashing, no crying out to God. Just him and his loved ones. Just like that he was gone. It seemed as if he was still sleeping.

I glanced into my grandfather's bony face and half-open eyes. Gone was the stress. His muscles were relaxed for the first time in a long time. So, just like that, in an instant, his life had come to an end.

The man who married Nonna, who gave life to his children, who had seen war and famine and poverty, and who struggled valiantly to realize his goal for himself and his family, was gone. All the toil and labor performed on the land, all the soil he and my father had tilled side by side. All gone, never to be done again by Nonno.

I was tired and hot.

"What did all he went through matter?" I thought long and hard about the silly things that always got my goat. "Why do all those trivial things matter when we're all going to finish like this?" I ran my fingers through my hair pulling it back away from my face as my mind continued to process the event. "It wasn't about all the material possessions, none of that comforts you in the end."

The sound of soft rubber heels patting the tiled floor materialized into a doctor who was called to the room to confirm the obvious. She listened for a heartbeat and placed a finger on the old man's wrist. Her straight, black, bowl-shaped haircut covered her eyes as she leaned down. She shook her head, her hair now swinging side to side. She conveyed a look of sorrow to everyone, her lip curling in the right hand corner creating a small crease in an otherwise smooth and tanned complexion. We all understood.

"I'm sorry," she said in a slight Filipino accent. She shrugged her shoulders as if to say there was nothing more that could be done.

I sat on the bed close to my grandfather's legs.

"Zio was…" I blocked out Maria's words and the conversation around me. "Maria…" Josephine's response faded out. I sat on the edge of the bed looking at my grandfather.

With Nonno now gone the wheels of strategy were moving as the siblings gathered to discuss how to best break the news to Martha.

"De (Tony's nickname for his younger brother), you go with Olivia and tell Martha." My dad spoke softly still holding his hand to his chin. He looked thin beneath his brown cotton shirt. His wispy graying hair floating out to the sides combined with his red, tired eyes to give him a defeated look.

"And while you're there, pick out a suit for Nonno," he instructed.

I stared down at my grandfather feeling a huge sense of loss and frustration. He had now left his children to deal with the mess he created by marrying this woman. This time however, the sense of loss beat out the resentment.

By the time everyone finally had their action plans, it was nine fifteen. I decided to leave with my aunt and uncle and make my way back home. The room's occupants said their goodbyes knowing that in a matter of a day, they would all be seeing one another again to send off our patriarch. I glanced over my shoulder one last time before going down the hall past the nurse's station and glimpsed at my grandfather through the open door.

"Goodbye," I whispered.

I opted to take the stairs rather than wait for the elevator. Passing the emergency room and its ten or so patients, I emerged into the dark night. I stopped just outside the entrance to call my mother.

"Hi."

"Charlie?" She seemed surprised to hear from me. "Oh, hi!"

A taxicab honked as I spoke.

"We're leaving the hospital now so Dad should be on his way soon."

"You know, I just think it's crazy that he's spent the entire day at the hospital."

My mother went on and on, not thinking about what she was saying. "Ma," I said, upset by the way this conversation was going and stopping her in her tracks. "Nonno died."

"Oh my God, Charlie, I…"

"I have to go and call Lisa." I took a deep breath, let out a sigh of frustration at my mother's ignorance and hung up. When I stopped to really think about it, I couldn't blame her. After all, my mother was just a product of her upbringing. What did she know about losing a father?

◆   ◆   ◆

With a gentle left turn, I drove into the brightly lit driveway. Lights from the house cast a warm glow onto the perfectly manicured lawn. Lisa waited in the living room. She had the front door open by the time I had made my way to the first step.

I recounted the events of the last few hours interspersed with sips of coffee Lisa had made while awaiting my arrival. I sat dumfounded. There was an inexcusably striking similarity between the scene now unfolding compared to one nineteen years earlier when it was my father at the kitchen table recounting Nonna's passing. Now here I was, playing the same part Dad did all those years ago.

17

The Eulogy

Echoes of coughs and sobs bounced off the marble walls of the mausoleum. The group of sixty family members and friends all looked in the same direction toward where a slab had been removed creating a gaping hole in the wall that housed my grandmother's casket. This same opening would now become my grandfather's resting place.

I was there physically, but my thoughts were reliving the events of the past few days. I had found out a lot about Nonno during the course of his wake from those who had a different view of him, than from those who saw his vulnerable side.

My eyes scanned the group of mourners.

"Brothers and sisters let us..."

The priest was saying his blessing over Nonno's casket. My swollen eyes came to rest on my cousins. Nonno was always particularly fond of his nieces. Zina most of all, and Maria Pia. It was obvious they had been the center of his universe, even more so that his own grandchildren. I accepted this and didn't mind. I had not been close to Nonno as was evidenced by the relatively few times I had visited him in recent years. It was a fact I regretted.

The events of the past few days swirled in my mind with tornadic force. I recalled all the conversations, and the opportunities they offered to learn a bit more about my grandfather from someone else's point of view.

◆   ◆   ◆

The room on the first floor of the funeral parlor was quite crowded with family and friends and the many paisani that came to pay their respects. Charles surveyed the scene from the doorway. It wasn't often he wore a suit, but when he did he looked quite dashing. The navy pinstripe was one of his favorites. He laughed to himself as he looked into the faces of those attending. The room was clearly demarcated. The old guard to the left, the new generation to the right.

The newer group consisting mostly of his cousins, was talking among themselves while the stoic crowd of older women opposite with their kerchiefs and rosaries, sat staring at them.

"Who are these people who think they can come here and judge others?" Charles thought and scowled. "Where were they when Nonno was alive?" His disdain was directed to only a few of those gathered, not to the masses.

"Hey Maria," he kissed his cousin and sat next to her in the second row of folding chairs. He sat on the end of the row so he could stretch his long legs and still have a good view of his grandfather bathed in soft light in one corner of the room. A red rosebud rosary was strung along the inner lid of the casket.

"My mother…"

He heard his cousin talking, but his eyes were fixed on the casket. "…had a dream that she was in a beautiful garden. As she entered, she saw two men."

"Who were they?" he asked. He loved listening to dreams, especially when they dealt with loved ones.

"Your grandfather's father and brother, the one who had died when he was hit by lighting," she said somberly.

Charles turned from the casket and scanned her face. The overhead lighting cast dark circles under her eyes. Maria Pia's bony cheek plates protruded from her smooth white face.

"I never knew Nonno had a brother who died," Charles said amazed. "Wow." He was captivated by the news his cousin had given him. He readjusted himself to face her, and crossed his right leg to rest on the left one.

"Yeah. He was working in the fields with Zio (as she referred to her uncle Charlie) and my father when a storm struck. Unable to find shelter, he was hit," she took a deep breath and sighed. "They carried his body, trying to find a place to stay until the storm passed. They did find a small abandoned barn, which they stayed in until it was safe," she said, pausing to take another breath.

Charles was mesmerized not so much by the news, but how Maria spoke. She was quiet, but the emotion in her voice was clear.

"So anyway," she gestured with her hands as if shooing a fly. "In my mom's dream, she went into the garden where everything was green and lush. They were preparing a feast, a celebration of sorts," she stopped.

"And…" Charles questioned, wanting to know how the dream ended.

"My mother asked if she could stay and they both said no. They told her she had to leave, that this was for someone else."

Charles' gaze momentarily shifted to the new guests who were now making their way toward the casket waiting their turn to kneel by Nonno.

"You know, your grandfather knew he was dying," Maria said out of the blue.

Her dark features were so much more evident in this room. Her thin, pale, long face was shockingly sallow against the blackness of her long straight hair. For someone so young, her eyes held the sorrow of a much older woman. She had lost her father a few years earlier, and now the last link to him, her uncle.

"How?" Charles said, squinting his eyes and shaking his head. "How did he know?"

◆　　　◆　　　◆

"Death is not an end, but a…"

The speech from the Filipino priest continued. As he spoke, I wondered when I would be called to give my speech. I was hoping I was ready, but suddenly I doubted my ability to keep it together. My thoughts were still on the conversation of a few days ago and why I was now standing waiting to speak.

◆　　　◆　　　◆

"Zio came by our house on his scooter the Thursday before he was admitted to the hospital," Maria's eyes were downcast. "I was crying."

"Why?" Charles said, totally stumped.

"He wanted someone to accompany him as he made his rounds saying goodbye to everyone. I stopped by Aunt Angelina first," she said. Maria never lifted her head as she spoke. "So you can imagine I was a basket case. There Zio is on his scooter riding through the streets of Astoria with me behind him, following him, crying hysterically."

Charles patted her shoulder. They both chuckled faintly at the thought. He saw a tear escape her eye.

"I had no idea that he knew," Charles said somberly. "I mean, I knew he had to know, he always mentioned death the last few months, but to really know, to have a sense that this is it."

Charles imagined himself knowing about his own demise and how he would have handled the news. "Probably not that bravely," he concluded.

He leaned forward experiencing an extreme sense of loss and sympathy for Nonno. His chin came to rest on the palm of his left hand. The prickly hairs of his goatee pinched his skin. He glanced over the black-suited shoulders of those in front of him to view Nonno resting in his flower-adorned casket.

A sudden series of motions caught Charles' eye. His uncle Diego was waving to him to come over. Charles was still melancholy over the entire discussion as he got up. His palms flattened against the tops of his knees as he got up slowly.

"Maria, thanks for telling me that story," he touched her shoulder. "Diego wants me, I'll talk to you later."

His cousin nodded.

Making his way to the front row on the opposite side of the small room, his uncle asked him, "Did you ever speak in public?"

"Of course!" he responded assuredly. "I'm a pro."

Charles really was quite a good speaker. One of his roles as a human resources manager was to give numerous training workshops to managers and staff. He enjoyed speaking. Charles also liked being the center of attention, a far cry from the introverted kid in grammar school and high school.

"Why do you ask?" the nephew shot back.

"Josephine doesn't want to give the eulogy. Do you want to do it?" Diego asked him.

Charles was intrigued now as he lowered himself into a kneel in front of his aunt and uncle.

"You don't want to do it, Jo?" he asked his aunt.

She smirked tightlipped and shook her head. Her black hair bobbed back and forth striking her pale white cheeks. Her features were so similar to Maria's.

Charles thought for a moment, hesitant to answer because he didn't know how he would react giving a eulogy. At the same time, he felt guilty because he really had not been the best grandson. But he was the oldest grandchild and Nonno's namesake.

"Okay," he said, without thinking about it any further. "Yeah, I'll do it."

Charles felt the pressure in his knees as he slowly got up.

"What did I just get myself into?" he thought as he took a seat along the wall. Lisa was sitting in front of him.

◆　　　◆　　　◆

"May the Lord Bless you, in the name of the Father and of the…"

The concluding blessing was being delivered. I gulped hard knowing that I would soon have to deliver the eulogy.

"Amen."

Thinking the service was over, some mourners started for the double glass doors of the mausoleum. Leading the charge was Martha. She no doubt wanted to get a head start to my parent's house and the buffet spread. She just didn't give a damn. She had caused so many problems for Nonno. The old saying, "An idle mind is the devil's workshop" rang true when it came to this woman. She had nothing to do with her time, but conjure up things that constantly amazed my family.

Uncle Diego ran over to the funeral director who was obviously not aware I was doing the eulogy. In a way I was somewhat relieved. Then I saw the director's head nod and look toward me.

◆   ◆   ◆

"I'm doing the eulogy," Charles informed his wife.

"What?" she seemed surprised. "Can you handle it?"

"I guess."

Lisa knew that even after nineteen years, Charles was still bent out of shape over losing his grandmother.

Nonno's casket was catty-cornered, directly diagonal from the door. Charles drew comfort from the many friends and family members that had joined them. He kept an eye on his father, concerned with how he was handling the stress of Nonno's death. Charles thought his father was doing surprisingly well talking with all the visitors from the company where he was employed. Even the owners of the company stopped by. This was just what his dad needed right now—conversation and distraction.

Josephine and Diego were the only ones sitting up front keeping vigil over Nonno. Tony had not sat by Nonno for more than two minutes since he arrived. He didn't like being up there staring at the lifeless body. He preferred to be talking, and Charles didn't blame him. However, Charles knew the ladies sitting in the third row did not approve of Tony's behavior. Their heads never moved, but they sat and watched.

The scene was reminiscent of Nonna's wake. The mourners here today were present then. They hadn't changed much, except for some additional weight and a bit more gray hair peeking out from their dark kerchiefs.

Charles couldn't help but laugh to himself. Here they sat once again playing the part that they were best suited for; looking mournful and passing judgment. Their eyes looked scornful at those who were smiling or chatting openly and casually. Their ignorance was to be mocked.

"Charlie," Diego called to him.

Once again Charles walked over to where his uncle sat.

"I started writing down a speech. You look it over and revise it, but try to keep it the same," he instructed his nephew, and handed him the piece of notebook paper.

"Oh," Diego continued. "The church will not allow us to do the eulogy at the Mass. It has to be done at the cemetery."

"What? Damn nothing ever comes easy for me," Charles said under his breath. It was just his luck that there would be a wrench in the whole process.

"This is ludicrous. We're supposed to be celebrating his life. That was the purpose of the Mass, no?" Charles told Lisa later on. "Yet, it was against the church's rules to allow eulogies, a bunch of bullshit, if you ask me. They were so quick to take Nonno's money though."

This was uncharacteristic for him. Charles was not normally so vocal about his contempt for the church since he had, up until recently, always had been its biggest defender. However, this incident sent him over the edge.

The morning of Nonno's burial, Charles paid a special visit to the rectory. He wanted to ask the Monsignor one last time if the 'no eulogy' rule could be lifted for Nonno. He went to ask this without the knowledge of anyone in his family. Charles thought he owed it to his grandfather to try one last time.

Charles passed the six-foot tool wrought iron fence, walked up to the rectory door and pressed the button on the intercom. His one short press did not bring any response. He was about to walk away when a voice came over the intercom. "Hello, can I help you?"

"Yes," Charles responded heading back toward the small slatted box hanging midway on the wall next to the rectory door. "I'd like to speak to Monsignor LoBrutto."

"This is he."

"Monsignor, my grandfather is being buried today and I was hoping to see if I could give the eulogy in church. It would mean a lot to us," Charles said, pleading his case.

"I'm afraid that will not be possible," the Monsignor's words were cold and unemotional. "For if I allowed one person to do it, I would need to allow everyone."

"I see."

"I'm sorry," the Monsignor said. His voice was insincere and patronizing.

Charles walked away. He was sure things would have been different if he had offered a donation of five hundred dollars. The Monsignor probably would have changed his tune. Money talked in this parish, but Charles wasn't about to offer them anything. Nonno had given enough to this church, putting a ton of change into those votive candles and weekly offerings. He walked back to his car and drove off to the funeral home.

This was always the hardest part of the process, saying the final goodbye. At his grandmother's funeral, Charles had completely come apart. Now, standing by Nonno's casket, he was crying again. He was taken aback by just how much his grandfather's passing affected him. He went downstairs to the bathroom. His eyes were green.

They left the funeral home and drove the short distance to the church, the procession passed by Nonno's house one last time. Charles blew his nose into a flimsy paper tissue. A knife went through his heart as he looked through the dark windows of the limo to the house that had been his oasis. He kept an eye on his father in the front passenger seat. His dad was taking this hard.

The limo pulled up in front the church. There was no conversation the entire way. The pallbearers removed the coffin from the silver hearse. The bronze rectangular box reflected the sun in all directions. Each of the metal corners was carved to depict religious scenes; the pieta, the last supper. That's all that was visible from Charles' vantage point.

The group walked up the five steps to the church following Nonno. The bells began tolling.

The family got as far as ten steps down the aisle before they were halted. The funeral director had disappeared behind the altar to the office with an envelope to give the Monsignor. They stood in the aisle behind the draped coffin waiting for someone to appear. It was an awkward moment.

"Diego, perche aspettiamo?" (Why are we waiting?) Olivia asked her husband. Her Borgettano accent showed through.

"Aunt Olivia," Charles said, grinning mischievously and squinting so his eyebrows came to a point right above his nose. "We're waiting here because the priest wants to make sure he has his money." Charles gestured, rubbing his thumb against his forefinger. His sarcasm and cynicism was not lost on her.

"Yeah," she laughed heartily, and patted her nephew's forearm. "Yeah, that'sa right, Charlie."

Charles knew his comment did not please his father who shot him a very disapproving look over his right shoulder. Tony turned to his brother who was standing in front of Charles. "I don't know who I take after, De." Charles and his aunt smirked. He looked devilish. He had not been eating well over the past few days and his face was gaunt. When the Monsignor finally emerged, Olivia and Charles looked at one another and laughed again.

Charles nudged his aunt. "Look," he said upon sighting the Monsignor, blatant sarcasm in his voice. "Here he comes. See how happy he is now that he got his money."

This whole ordeal had left such a bad taste in Charles' mouth. He knew Tony had taught him and his siblings about going to church to pray, but then getting out. "Don't get involved with the church," Tony had told them. For someone as religious as he, it was a strange thing to say. But now Charles understood what his dad meant.

◆   ◆   ◆

"Ladies and gentlemen, I have been told that Charles' grandson, Charles would like to say a few words," the barrel-chested funeral director announced. His voice boomed through the cavernous interior. The departing entourage led by the tightly wrapped Martha, stopped and turned back.

I glanced around the 'condominium,' the name I gave these structured mausoleums. The smell infiltrated my senses; a mixture of moisture and formaldehyde with flowers thrown in for good measure. I stood in front of the gaping hole in the wall containing the coppery metallic box housing my grandmother's coffin.

"Hi, Nonna," I whispered.

Had she originally been buried in this wall, I would now be looking at her actual casket, but she was first interred in the ground at St. Raymond's in the Bronx. In early 1993, my grandfather had decided to get this 'condo' at St. Michael's mausoleum and he moved her body that year. Reposing next to Nonna was Uncle Angelo, Nonno's brother who lay next to his in-laws. Above Nonna, the fathers of two of my friends lay; Corrado's dad Anthony, and Maria G.'s father.

We had grown up on the same block as Maria G. She lived only a few doors down from our house in Astoria. They were the nicest people you'd ever want to know. I missed all those younger years, and often thought of the old block and the people we knew there like the Giarratano's; people from the 'old town' who always returned to Italy each summer. In an instant I remembered the one summer Maria and her family left for Italy. I had said goodbye to Maria and her dad from the stoop of his backyard. The sky was ablaze in navy and hot pink as the sun set.

Glancing above the heads of those gathered, all appearing like one large black ink spot through my moist eyes, I began.

"My grandfather's life reads like a good book, all of it true. He was born in New York City in 1913, while his father and mother were still in America."

The sound of my voice was deafening as it echoed off the marble slabs. My ears hurt. It was as if I wasn't the one talking, but rather someone from far away over a microphone.

"His father wanted to make enough money and return to Italy, which they did when my grandfather was three."

◆   ◆   ◆

Charles' great-grandfather Antonio was a tough man who earned most of his money by playing cards in the bars and cafes. He had come to the United States on a few occasions, one time aboard the ship Calabria, which left Palermo on July 13, 1912 and arrived into New York on July 29, 1912 where he stayed with a cousin in Manhattan.

◆   ◆   ◆

"Although he completed his formal education in the third grade, my grandfather never stopped learning. His father enlisted him to work on the land when my grandfather was only nine-years-old. He worked full time and made the land look like a garden. My grandfather's will and desire for a better life made him look beyond this small piece of land."

I bit my lip to control the sobs that were beginning to form deep within me. I stopped to regain my composure. Lifting my left hand and placing it upon the casket, I continued.

"He wanted to come to the United States at the age of sixteen. This request was denied by his father who worried that if my grandfather left that would set a precedent his other brothers would follow. Who would work the land then? Soon after getting married to my grandmother…"

I turned my head to acknowledge my grandmother who lay just beyond the hole in the wall. I was crying now. I soon realized that so were most of the mourners. I took a hard swallow and continued.

"Soon after getting married to Nonna, he was called into the Army to serve in World War Two. He never lost sight of his goal to come to America. After the war and after years of red tape, he made the dream a reality in 1958. At the age of forty-five, he moved his family to begin a new life."

My chest was tight.

"My grandfather was a pioneer. As someone who is in the business world, I'll use a phrase we talk about a lot, 'thinking out of the box.' My grandfather did that. But the story doesn't end there. It would be too easy. After coming to America and getting a job with Sunshine Biscuits, he began sponsoring his family to come to America; his in-laws, his brother. The process continued until all who wanted to come here were able. My grandfather opened the door for others. He gave back!"

I was a bit calmer now, and thought that my eulogy was flowing rather nicely.

"He raised a family of three successful children who have gone on to raise families of their own. He was always concerned with providing for his family. Many of you may recall how an accident twenty-three years ago almost claimed his life, but it didn't. His will was strong, and to him, this was a setback, not the end. God gave us all this extra time. His children, grandchildren, nieces, nephews and so on, to get to know him even better."

My composure was short-lived as I once again found myself having to pause because of my crying. My sobs were getting a bit more audible now and I became keenly aware of the pressure that was building in my head from my efforts to suppress my tears. I was deathly afraid of completely losing it with the next paragraph. I never once looked up at the group.

"I was just asked the other day, what was one memory I have of my grandfather. For me, it was the time he and I traveled to Italy back in 1982. After getting off to a rocky start with my grandfather yelling and waving his crutch at the flight attendant as to why we didn't have window seats, it turned out to be a pretty good trip."

By this time everyone was laughing. They knew Nonno all too well. It was exactly like my grandfather to be stubborn and argumentative.

"But there was one moment for me, a moment that defined for me the true essence of my grandfather. It was one day of the tour when we visited Pisa, practically eighteen years ago today. It was a day like today."

I motioned my right hand upward, and turned my face to the blue sky visible through the glass skylight directly above us.

"The tour group was going to climb the stairs of the tower to the observation deck. Being fifteen at the time, I was content to watch the tower from a distance, but not my grandfather. He was there and he was going to climb it!"

More chuckles erupted from the group.

"I just remember him climbing the narrow stairs with his one crutch supporting him. Everyone in the group was blown over by his determination. He had won the admiration and respect of all that day, including myself.

"This moment defined for me who Nonno was. He wasn't happy just seeing things from afar. He needed to be in the middle of the action, and I see the same will in his children, a lot in me, and even in my three-year old."

My chest became heavy. I could no longer contain the sobbing.

I slowly started to unravel as I started the next sentence.

"So," my voice cracked. "Here we've come to the final chapter of his life…"

I paused. Just totally and unashamedly crying now. I looked down at my feet, which were spotted with tears.

I glanced over to the metal legs of the scaffold holding the coffin, lifted my head and rested my left hand on Nonno's coffin. I heard sniffles throughout the crowd but dared not look. I tried concentrating on how polished the coffin felt—cool and smooth to the touch.

"And what a life it has been. His was a life that saw poverty, hard work, death…things that would break most people. His was also a life filled with goals and determination. He saw his goals realized. So, as we close this book, Nonno would often, and proudly, call me Ciali 2 (Nonno wrote my name this way in many of the cards I received), and refer to himself as Ciali 1."

I could no longer go on. My sobs were so bad and deep that my face and chest hurt. My head was pounding from squinting and the tightening of the muscles around my cheeks and forehead. My memories of hearing Nonno call me Ciali 2 were painful.

I looked out over the heads of the group without looking at any one particular individual. Sobs were coming from every direction.

"So Nonno," I cried, looking down at his casket, which was hazy from the tears in my eyes. "From Ciali 2 to Ciali 1 and from your entire family, we'll miss you and we love you. And although you may be gone, your spirit, values, and determination will always live within us."

It was over.

I was done.

No sooner had I let the last word out, than the emotional energy I held within me spewed forth along with a deep wail. I went over and hugged Lisa, who had her back to me and was crying just as uncontrollably. She couldn't bear to watch me as I spoke. Her eyes were swollen and red. We hugged one another and cried, pouring tears onto each others shoulders. Soon, the two of us became four as we were soon joined by Zina and Maria Pia.

"Thank you so much Charlie for that," Zina sobbed, hugging me. "Thank you."

I was surprised at the emotional toll this speech took on me. I honestly did not think I would react in such a demonstrative manner. I did love my grandfather and losing him meant I was losing the last real grandparent I had. Now there was no Nonna and no Nonno. That generation had passed. No longer would I see him on the streets of Astoria. No longer would I be able to stop by his house if I wanted to.

I glanced to my dad who was way over on the other side of the group. His eyes too, were red as he was comforted by Josephine and Diego.

With the eulogy complete, this chapter was closed.

18

Unexpected Treasure

"So, when did Nonna and Nonno get married?" I asked my dad.

My father stared into his coffee cup. His forefinger and thumb played lightly with the silver spoon immersed in the tan brew creating little waves within the cup. I sensed he did not immediately know the answer.

His forehead was lined like sheet music. From the tilt of my dad's head, his downward looking eyes and my view of his bald spot, I couldn't help but think how much he looked like St. Anthony. All joking aside, I was concerned about him. As the days following Nonno's death turned into weeks, he looked more tired and aged.

Clank. The spoon hit the side of the thick porcelain mug.

He glanced at Gabriella, Lisa, and I and placing both hands on the flower-decked tablecloth rose from his seat, his hands supporting his thin body. He never seemed to gain an ounce and the polo shirts he wore (usually shades of gray or beige), even though they were size small, always seemed to be too big on him. For as long as I could remember, he was the same weight.

Without a word, he turned and walked down the narrow hallway to his bed-room. With the exception of his brown pants, there was no color to speak of in the corridor, just beige as far as the eye could see. No pictures hung on the walls. The only contrast to the ecru painted surface was the wainscot and eye-level thermostat. Even the door off to right of the hall was painted in the same ecru color.

This was quite a contrast to the vivid colors used in my house. I hated the blandness of 'off-white' and laughed at the comedic sense of the word. Having lived in our house for close to five years now, I shocked Lisa when I decided to paint our foyer a beautiful, bright yellow.

I thought the regal looking color highlighted the gilded frame of the pictures and mirror hanging on the wall. One picture was a Madonna with Child in a five by eight frame next to the curved arch of the entry. That picture always brought me a sense of peace and tranquility, (I liked using the French version of the word 'tranquilité') something I needed desperately in my own life.

Then there were the two kissing angels visible to anyone upon entering our warm home. Lastly, an ornately carved gold-framed mirror hung from the largest of the walls in the foyer.

I hated looking into this mirror, especially on days when I knew I didn't look good. Nonetheless, each time I exited or entered the house, my eyes were always drawn to it. Depending on my mood, my reflection was either a warm smile or a grimacing, condescending stare.

The remainder of the house also exuded warmth with color. A deep crimson adorned the lower half of our dining room walls, while the upstairs bath was graced in lemony yellow. It was the kind of yellow that elicited thoughts of an early spring morning with sun shining brightly in periwinkle blue skies, and white sheer panels billowing in a light breeze. I liked the color I had chosen for this room and for all the rooms in our house.

No sooner had my dad disappeared through the bedroom door to the left of the hall than I, almost reluctantly, placed my coffee cup on the table and joined him. I loved coffee, especially when I was sitting outside on my deck watching the blue of the early evening sky become navy, the cool air hitting my cheeks, the warm cup in my hands.

By now my father was on a search through desk drawers, a bookcase, and finally the room's adjoining closet. I could make out his silhouette, thanks to the light coming in from windows alongside the small closet. At last he emerged with a weathered envelope and emptied the contents of the faded yellow treasure chest onto his bed.

"What's all that?" I inquired.

A smile came across the whisker stubble of his face.

"It's all their important papers," he said. "Let's try to find when they were married, see if there's a marriage certificate in here."

I looked down at the pile of papers, tattered and yellow edged, and began to sift through them. Each piece of paper I took from the flowered bedspread held an amazing but poignant reminder of my grandparent's history. I unfolded one paper after the other amazed at the amount of information before me.

Gabriella was growing restless and her whines were becoming more audible from the living room.

"Why not just take the whole envelope home and see what you find," my father said.

The moment he said those words, I felt as if someone had handed me a million dollars.

I responded without hesitation. "Wow. Okay, I'll bring it back Monday."

With one scoop of my hand, I hurriedly placed all the papers back into the envelope, all the while relishing the thought of going through each one while in the privacy of my own home.

I held the envelope close to my dark navy short-sleeved shirt, and once I arrived at the car, dropped it into the soft leather of the passenger seat.

No sooner had we driven off when Lisa, who was sitting in the back seat with Gabriella, extended her bare arm over the front seat and snatched the envelope. She kept an eye on our very active three-year-old and opened the envelope. I had wanted to get home and be the first to look at the contents.

I felt that pit in my stomach, the same one when someone read the Sunday newspaper before I did. I grew impatient and resentful. After all, this was my grandparents' information and I should be the one to go through it first.

For once though, I kept my mouth shut. At a stoplight, Lisa picked out one paper at a time from the envelope, unfolded the document and revealed what it was. The first item was a settlement letter from when my grandfather was hit by the car. This was the final paper awarding him damages from his suit against the drunk driver and his employer.

The next piece was a notarized letter translated in English recording the birth of someone I did not recognize. Lisa folded it back to its three-inch square size and proceeded onto the next document, a very crisp piece of paper with a single crease going down its five-inch length. It had a picture of Nonna on it. It was her Naturalization certificate dated December 30, 1963.

The photo of Nonna was the same one used for her headstone when she was buried in St. Raymond's Cemetery (the same photo was also used for the cover of this book).

The signal light turned green.

I held the Naturalization paper in my hands spanning the steering wheel. After a sharp left turn onto the service road of Grand Central, I managed to grab the right corner of the document and hand it over my shoulder to Lisa. She folded it and pulled out the next item.

"Wow," she exclaimed. In the rearview mirror I saw she held a passport. I could see her eyes scanning it.

"What do you have there?" I asked, impatiently looking back to the road, making sure no asshole was cutting in front of me.

"Your grandmother's passport." She held the document open, her blonde hair dancing lightly over the surface of the page like marionettes on strings. She continued studying the same page.

"Let me see." I reached back to grab it at the next red light and opened the navy blue cover. I flipped through the entry visa pages. All were empty. Never stamped. I finally came to Nonna's photo. It looked recent. Her hair was pulled back by a clip of some sort. Funny, I didn't remember my grandmother ever wearing her hair that way.

Glancing up real quick, I wiped strands of hair from my eyes and face. I noticed the light was still red. Glancing back down, I looked at the date of issuance—January 14, 1981. I stared at the date for what seemed like an eternity and remembered how much Nonna wanted to travel to Italy.

◆   ◆   ◆

July of 1981 proved how hot the summers in New York could be and this particular Sunday was no exception. Despite the fact it was only six forty-five in the morning, the humidity pressured Charles awake.

Charles felt the stinging in his toe almost immediately upon placing his bare foot on the cool linoleum floor. He had been suffering with an ingrown toenail on his big right toe. He hadn't cared for it properly and it had become so painful he could hardly walk, let alone spend an entire day strawberry picking with his family as was the case today.

The weekends during the summer months were predictable, starting with getting up early and making lunches for the day's excursion. Since Tony hated any meal remotely associated with fast food, he insisted on making sandwiches at home to take along in the cooler.

Charles scratched at his matted hair as he limped from his room. He entered the kitchen to find his father in front of an assembly line of cold cuts, Italian bread, lettuce, and sliced tomatoes all sprawled on the dining room table.

Tony took his eyes from the loaf of Italian bread he had just sliced to glance at the youngster. "Would you like ham or turkey?" he asked his half-awake son.

"Ham," came the half-hearted response.

A good three slices of the pink meat decorated the bottom half of a six-inch wedge of bread. Tony added two tomato slices, a handful of lettuce, and completed the sandwich with a slice of bread on top.

He held the edge of a roll of foil, pulled it quickly out to arms length and in an instant, sliced it on the sharp teeth along the edge of the box. A wrap of the silvery aluminum finished off each sandwich.

Today the family was going out with their friends Sal and his children. Sal and Tony had been friends even before they arrived in the US back in 1959. They were so different. Sal cussed a lot when he came to visit, which often made Tony cringe. To Tony, the word "damn" was a bad word. So, it was often comical to see Tony's expressions when Sal talked and talked.

On these weekends, it was the same ritual; friends and family would meet at a gas station at seven in the morning. After driving for close to two hours on the Long Island Expressway to Riverhead, they would spend the next few hours picking strawberries, apples or whatever happened to be in season. After picking a few bushels, the group would call it a day and drive off to Wildwood Park on the Northern tip of Long Island for lunch. For the most part, Charles enjoyed these outings, but today was a different story.

Charles' toe hurt terribly all week. The skin was inflamed where his nail had grown under the skin. What made it worse was the irritation caused by the toe next to it, rubbing up against the sore part. Charles had tried to clip the nail, but to no avail. Greenish, oozing puss was not a good sign either.

"I don't want to go today!"

Charles' insistence drew ire from his father who in a moment of anger took his son's right sneaker, which had been sitting near the dishwasher, and proceeded to cut off the whole toe part. The dark navy blue top hit the floor as the teen stared in disbelief. With the entire toe of the shoe (with the exception of the sole) officially amputated, his blue sneaker looked ridiculous on his white-socked foot.

With no other pair of shoes around, and not wanting to draw attention to his ridiculous plight, Charles got creative, which he was anyway. He went into his bedroom and quickly tried changing into socks of different colors, trying to see which would be less conspicuous. He finally settled on a pair of brown dress socks.

He emerged from his bedroom and stood in the kitchen. His shorts, cut-up sneaker and mid-calf length brown dress socks made quite a fashion statement. By this time the young boy was angry and determined as ever not to go with his family, and made this point quite clear to his father as he proceeded past the beige walls of the kitchen and headed out the backyard door.

"I'll be at Nonna's," he exclaimed defiantly, and walked down the alleyway, brown socks and all. It was only seven thirty in the morning.

Nonna was up, and as always was glad to see her grandson. She sympathetically listened to his tale of woe, and as the case whenever she heard bad news, scrunched her face a bit and after a tsk-tsk said a Bedra Madre (Blessed Mother).

Later that morning Nonna prepared something to put on his toe. In a small saucepan, she mixed olive oil, garlic and bread until all the ingredients were hot and liquefied. The sizzle of the oil scared Charles. He thought the concoction would burn the skin right off his appendage. Rolling the mixture up in gauze she said, "This izza fromma Italy," and placed a small amount of the stew in a white handkerchief and placed it directly on his toe.

Charles had noticed something pensive in her voice and her demeanor. After getting over the initial stinging from the hot blend, he felt the heat and the ingredients working their magic. Nonna just sat by him looking down at his toe, which by this time was ruby red.

The stifling heat of the room was uncomfortable for him, made even worse by the plastic slipcovers of the gold sofa. Charles was becoming one with the plastic as he felt himself melting into it. The sweat was beading on the backs of his knees.

"Italia," she whispered softly. Her mind was still wandering. She was thinking about Italy, perhaps pondering the cruel reality that she was never going to have the chance to visit one last time. Charles had seen that look in her eyes many times before. Like those times at the airport when the family saw his grandfather off on one of his many visits to Sicily to check on his dry parcel of land. These trips to the airport were vivid and clear to him.

Charles jumped at any chance to go to the airport and he remembered standing in the waiting area of the gate in the International Arrivals building while they said their buon viaggio to Nonno. Overhead hung a Plexiglas sign with the unmistakable logo of Alitalia emblazoned on it, a red triangle surrounded by the green letter 'a.' His grandmother had the same look now as she did when she had said all those goodbyes at the airport.

◆   ◆   ◆

I fingered the passport. My forefinger glided over the grainy cover and I chuckled to myself ever so lightly remembering the events later that same afternoon.

◆   ◆   ◆

Drrriiinnng!

The phone called for attention.

Nonna gripped the walker. Her arms shook as she strained to lift herself from the sofa. The flesh at the bottom of her arms sagged and moved from side to side as she made her way through the doors to her bedroom, her nightgown light and breezy around her.

"Ello," she said into the black receiver. "Che Giuseppina?" (Hi, what is it Josephine?) She gingerly sat on the edge of her bed as she spoke.

From the rest of the conversation, Charles could make out that his aunt was coming over for a barbeque.

"Sure, ehh, okay, bye."

Charles heard the clunk of the black receiver.

"Ciali," she called.

"Yeah, Nonna?"

He raised himself off the sofa. His clothing peeled away from the sweaty plastic causing sweat stains across the back of his navy blue shorts. He joined her in the bedroom. She was rummaging through the middle drawer of her dresser.

Nonna kept her furniture meticulous. The brown, highly-polished dresser shined brilliantly in the midmorning sun flooding through the lace-paneled windows. A large mirror ran the length of the legged piece reflecting a pair of ornate vases adorning each end of the dresser. The vases were no more than twelve inches high with brightly painted flowers and decorations with two handles painted in turquoise. Between the two vases was a bisque statue of the Virgin Mother. Its faint, almost dull colors, brought symmetry to the placement.

Nonna's hands were now buried in one of the drawers searching under neatly folded clothes, navy and black for the most part with a thin slice of beige. She found what she was looking for, a small navy blue purse.

"Josephine viene per barbeque," she said, as she reached into the purse advising her grandson that Josephine was coming over for a barbeque.

She brought out some bills, a ten and a twenty. "You go a to Key Food and buy chickena, e qualcosa." (Somethings.)

"Okay," he dutifully responded. But then he remembered his predicament. Before he could think up a plan for how he was going to go to the store with his sneaker ripped in half and brown socks exposed, he was out the door.

As he went through the gate of the front yard, once again his resourcefulness and creativity set in. He walked on the side of the street where there were no people. If he saw someone crossing into his path, Charles simply readjusted his steps and walked in the street. Before he knew it, he had completed the four-block trip.

But now there was a new set of issues to tackle. He walked through the store quickly so no one would detect the deformity, but now, having picked out the selection of meat, he had to endure the more difficult task of standing in the checkout line. He was at the mercy of a pretty long line even though it was supposedly the Express Check-out. As he stood waiting his turn, he strategically crossed his legs covering his bad foot by resting the other one on top of it.

Finally, after what seemed like an eternity, Charles had reached the check out counter, and after paying, took the back exit leading to the parking lot. There were less people there. He duplicated the same game plan back to his grandmother's house.

"Whew," the chubby teen let out a victory sigh when he entered the safety of the gate.

◆   ◆   ◆

I glanced up. "Red light still?" I thought to myself.

As opposed to looking back down at the passport, I chose to glance out onto the road before me. The cars whizzed by as I sat, my eyes fixed on a certain point of road just above my black leather steering wheel.

◆   ◆   ◆

Charles placed the groceries on the kitchen table and handed Maria the leftover change. She went into her bedroom to put the change back in its secret hiding place.

"Ciali," she called over her shoulder to her eldest grandchild still in the kitchen pulling groceries from the coarse brown bag and lining them neatly on the clean white surface of the tabletop. He stopped unpacking to join her. She extended her arm and handed him a rolled up bill. Charles looked at her questioning.

"This izza for you."

Charles saw it was a ten dollar bill.

"Howwa you say," she looked around the room for the right words. "This izza fromma tha bottom offa my heart."

Charles nodded his head and clenched his lower lip beneath his large front teeth.

"I lovva you," she said. Her eyes bore deep into her grandson's. Her features, especially her eyes, were dark and piercing, and never showed anything but the love she had in her heart.

Standing next to her, he could not bring himself to say those three words back.

"Me too, Nonna," was all he could faintly manage. He hugged her. It was all he could muster, and as he patted his grandmother's back, Charles could not understand

why it was so difficult for him to say 'I love you' back. He surely did love her, but why he could not utter the words remained a mystery to him.

When Josephine arrived for dinner later on that afternoon, they barbequed the chicken and hot dogs Charles had bought. They ate on the round, white vinyl table on the little patch of perfect cement in the backyard amid the grapevines and fig trees. Charles recounted the day's events that brought laughter from everyone, especially Nonna. It was good for him to see her laugh.

◆   ◆   ◆

The light turned green.

Through tear-filled eyes I managed to drive, still holding the passport between my fingers, while both hands grasped the steering wheel. I managed a glance down at the document every now and then.

"Charlie, you've got to get a grip," my wife reprimanded me.

My fingers rubbed across the vinyl cover. I couldn't help but think that Nonna had once touched this very item. I never knew she had gotten a passport.

"Why did she get a passport in the first place? And why in 1981?" I thought. "Maybe she was planning on taking that trip to Italy she always spoke about." My heart grew heavy. I could feel the tightness in my chest. Today was one of those days. At the bottom of the page there was something, or rather something *not* there. The passport was never signed.

I couldn't look at the document anymore for fear that I wouldn't be able to see the road thanks to all the tears in my eyes. They dripped slowly down my chin and then onto my neck, tickling as they slid down; darkening the navy color of my shirt. The highway ahead became blurry and I quickly wiped the salty liquid away from my eyes and mouth.

"Can I see the envelope again?" I asked Lisa. We were finally home and I opened the sliding glass doors to the deck. I took a seat on one of the white plastic chairs at the backyard table and spread the papers and forms onto the sea blue vinyl tablecloth with swimming fish. The colorful backdrop was in stark contrast to the yellow and white papers.

"After all that, this is all there is left," I said aloud.

Lisa was in the kitchen and couldn't hear me. I stared at the remnants of my grandparents lives neatly wrapped in an eight-by-four envelope. This was all that remained. I noticed a sharply creased and obviously old letter. I unfolded it. The document was in Italian. It was a passenger ticket for the *Saturnia*. That was the ship my father, Nonna, Diego, and Josephine sailed in on their journey from Sicily to the United States in 1959.

The cost of passage was typed in red, block letters. It was the kind of type that came from a really old typewriter. I pictured some guy in a gray suit at the shipping office sitting in front of a black monstrosity using his bony fingers to poke and peck the keys.

Passage for the four of them was six hundred thirty six dollars. That money represented at least a few good years of savings from their daily journeys to towns to sell their harvest. I couldn't fathom what it must have been like for them to save all that money. My mind raced as I thought of the sacrifices they must have made, the things they gave up. A sense of guilt overcame me, a feeling I knew all to well.

There was always an element of guilt in whatever I did despite the fact that I only had the best intentions. I pondered the cost of my relatives' ticket in relation to my luxury German sports sedan. I felt absolutely selfish that I was leasing a car with a monthly payment more than the price of their travel document to a better life.

Things seemed too easy, even with the griping about office politics, long hours, meetings, etcetera. No matter how much it seemed that I didn't care about where I came from, I now realized I cared a great deal. I had never forgotten the stories my dad told me growing up. There was no way to block out the hardships my family and the generations before me endured, to get their piece of the pie. Driving a sedan that few could afford was not going to make me escape my history.

My father always told me to save, no matter how much money I made. "It's not how much you make, but how you spend it." His advice resonated in my head as I pictured him speaking these words of wisdom on more than one occasion.

Even though I was successful by most standards, especially within my family, it was the duty of my father to always be concerned for me. That concern was evident when I purchased my home. After looking for more than a year, Lisa and I found the perfect brick saltbox colonial in a small community. We wanted to show my parents the home and had chosen also to garner their approval.

I drove them to the house one evening. We pulled up front and parked across the very narrow, one-way street. I glanced out the window of my gray coupe and noticed how the house glowed warmly from the inside. It seemed the owners had turned on the lights in almost every room in preparation for our visit.

We all got out of the car. The soft, incandescent lighting proved inviting in the darkness of the autumn evening.

"This is it?" my father asked Lisa.

He seemed stunned as his eyes swept the expanse of brick from one side of the house to the other. The symmetrical black-shuttered windows framing the center-hall entrance of the home exuded an air of distinction and originality.

"Yep," she said. "This is it."

I stood behind my dad smiling to himself, thinking that if the home's first impression astounded my dad, just think of how the rest of the family would react. I was big on impressing.

Even my grandfather seemed concerned about our purchase. In the first few years after moving in, he always made a point to ask me how the house was and how we were doing. Nonno always made sure to tell me 'be careful.' After a while he stopped asking feeling secure his grandson was doing okay.

But I knew where he was coming from. Both my grandfather and my dad saw how bad things could be when there wasn't any money around to support a family. It was not something they wanted their younger family members to experience.

I folded the ticket, or *biglietto*, as was written across the top, making sure the piece of paper was creased in the same way as when I opened it. No sooner was this task completed than I once again reached for the passport and opened it to the first page. I took note of the issue date and Nonna's photo. She seemed tired in the photo, her hair a bit grayer than I remembered. Again I thought of the unfamiliar way it was pulled back. It looked as if a clip had held it together, out of sight of the camera.

The irony of having been issued a passport in January, the same month her cancer had come back with a vengeance, did not escape me. A sinking feeling of guilt permeated me—not that it ever left me.

I sat alone under the cover of the iron awning staring out over the green grass of the yard and upward to the trees that touched the blue canopy of the sky beyond my patch of land.

The front of my shirt was drenched with an endless stream of tears, as was often the case whenever I thought of my grandmother. I wished she were alive today to see her great-granddaughter, to visit us in our home, to see the man I had become, and to know that she was proud of me.

Professionally, I was happy. I had finally reached that point in my life where I felt a modicum of success—paying the mortgage, supporting a family, traveling—it seemed like I was able to do it all. And best yet, not have to worry about money. My driven nature and desire to succeed had finally paid off. I knew that if I had to pick a character flaw of mine, it would be that I tired easily and became bored of the same old thing. Monotony was synonymous with death for me. Lisa often commented that she was surprised I was still married to her, the same woman I had known for eighteen years.

While I knew Nonna would have been proud of me, I wondered if she would really have cared about all the material stuff. In my heart, I knew the answer.

◆   ◆   ◆

Saturday, August 7, 1978 started out like a usual summer day; very hot and humid. Having spent a week at a lakeside retreat on Lake Vanare about eleven miles southwest of Lake George, it was time to return home. The morning found Tony packing the family car.

Something nagged at Charles, telling him he wouldn't be back to these log cabins. Each of these large wooden houses bore a different name: The Mountainview, The LakeView, The Beachview, and so on. There were seven efficiency units total, all very like a home away from home, but with a beach and the smell of cedar wafting through the air.

For Barbara, it was probably no vacation at all. One of the first things she did whenever they arrived was go to the local supermarket and load up on groceries. Tony would not allow them to eat at a fast food joint. No matter how much the three children pleaded to eat out, he always responded, "Never mind, we'll eat a good dinner at home." The long, five-hour ride home was unbearable in the two-door Ventura. Maria and Charles sat with their knees bent the entire ride, except for one or two stops to go to the bathroom. Mark was the only one able to sit comfortably.

Packing for their annual road trip was a comedic adventure in itself. Tony, unlike conventional travelers, didn't believe in using suitcases. His thing was to pack everything in plastic bags, fit as many into the trunk as possible, and then line the floor of the backseat. Leaving home was extra special since Tony would never pack the car in the morning. "What if the neighbors saw we were leaving?" So, instead, he resorted to heading out after dark when people were no longer out, and load the car. This way in the morning all they had to do was get in, let his tall lanky son get as comfortable as possible with knees practically at his chin, and head off.

With no air conditioning in the sky blue sports sedan, Tony kept the only two operable front windows open the entire ride. This often meant uninvited guests in the form of a bee or wasp joining them for the ride. Tony only pulled over after Charles or his sister screamed bloody hell.

Charles gazed out the triangular rear window and felt the heat of the late morning sun on his bare cheeks. The combination of heavy summer traffic and the smoky friction of rubber tires on the hot pavement caused a grimy haze just above the roadway. Country music created a soft background for his parents' discussions.

There was no FM on the radio, another extra Tony had no use for, so the occupants were at the mercy of the country or rock stations on the AM dial. A news announcement followed some whiny male singer crying about his horse, Wildfire.

"In Rome today, thousands of mourners flocked to St. Peter's Square to pay their respects to Pope Paul VI and gaze upon his body lying in state."

"Dad, turn this louder," Charles excitedly said. For once there was something on the radio he wanted to hear.

Tony adjusted the knob as the announcer continued.

"Due to the high heat in the Italian capital, the pope's body had started to decompose and needed to be treated with additional formaldehyde."

"Huh," Charles said softly to himself.

After exiting off the Triboro Bridge, the first stop the family made was to stop at Nonna's. Charles had bought her a cedar wood mail holder, which he was eager to give her. In addition, he wanted desperately to get out of the car, even if her house was only two minutes before theirs.

They all got out and climbed the stairs to the front door, joining up in the small kitchen before going outside. Nonna's backyard was a perfect haven; good next-door neighbors and long rows of vegetables planted on either side of the long middle walkway separating the two garden areas into two perfect rectangles.

Nonno maintained his grapes on scaffolding of metal pipes welded together. Like the radiators and steam pipes inside the house, these were painted the same silvery color. There was a nice patch of concrete perfectly maintained where Nonna kept the plastic lawn chairs or the occasional chaise lounge.

The shade of the grape canopy provided seclusion and a much needed harbor from the sun during the warmer months. A good cup of coffee from Nonna's chrome percolator was a nice treat for Charles and the family on those summer evenings when he watched the sky change to darker and deeper hues and enjoyed a cooling breeze against his bare arms and legs.

His long white knee socks with blue and red stripes at the top protected his calves. Although still in his early teens, Charles had been enjoying coffee since slicing his hand and receiving stitches back in 1974, when he was only in second grade. That was a traumatic evening for him.

◆   ◆   ◆

With one eye on the television and the other on the water glasses he held in his hands, Charles set the dinner table.

His pesky brother and sister were seated next to one another, not helping, but doing all they could to annoy him. Like mosquitoes buzzing in his ear, they spoke and laughed to one another looking at their older brother at various times. They had picked up the silverware he had just set down. Mark was the first to begin scraping a knife against a fork, as if he had two sticks in his hand trying to make fire. If there was one noise in this world that drove Charles crazy, that was it.

"Stop it Mark!"

The older sibling's request went unheeded by his sandy haired, big eyeglass-wearing brother. Instead, he continued grinding the two utensils together producing a sound akin to fingernails on a blackboard. Charles tried to ignore the painfully irritating sounds and continued to place the drinking glasses one by one near each of the dishes. The water glasses were small with red and yellow flowers adorning the circumference. Charles held one of them in his right hand preparing to place it on the table. His palm covered the open top.

The phone rang and Barbara went to answer it. Danny, her brother who she hadn't spoken to in years was on the line. By this point Charles' agitation over the scraping of the silverware got the best of him. His boiling point had reached the limit. "Stop it! I said stop," he yelled.

He slammed the glass down so hard that the fragile container shattered.

Searing pain pierced his hand and ran the length of his right arm. Charles looked down. He turned his palm over with his left hand and surveyed the damage. The wound scribed a semicircle across his palm just below his fingers. The meat from the inside of his hand protruded out and above the cut. Charles stretched his forefinger to push it back where it belonged. He could see clear through to the bone.

"Oh my God! What did I do?"

Barbara talked on, just looking at her son in disbelief as she continued the conversation with her brother. Charles couldn't help but think how his uncle had picked a fine night to call.

Charles grabbed a dishtowel, quickly wrapped his hand, and paced up and down the hallway from the dining room to the front door, repeatedly passing his mother on the phone.

"Oh my God. Oh my God," he repeated over and over as he continued his frantic pacing. Drops of blood from the saturated towel made perfect dots on the stone patterned linoleum. It took only a minute before the dishtowel was completely red. He raced back to the kitchen for another cloth dropping the used one to the floor and waited anxiously for his dad to arrive home from work.

The bleeding was starting to subside. He carefully removed the green and beige floral towel to expose the wound. The skin around the gash was like ricotta—the way fingertips get when you stay in a warm bath for too long.

"I don't have to go to the hospital, right?" Charlie asked as soon as his father arrived home.

Tony peered closely at the crevice in his son's hand. It was at least three-quarters of an inch deep and by this time absolutely bloodless. His father hurried to the dining table and grabbed the jug of wine closest to his chair and poured it right onto the cut, using the wine as a disinfectant. For Charlie, the pain was intense as the alcohol seared through his hand.

"Owwwwwww!"

Barbara, who by this time was off the phone, leapt up from the table as the wine splattered all over the dining room floor.

"Tony, what are you doing?" She grabbed a towel and threw it onto the ruby red soaked floor. She used the slipper on her foot to wipe the towel back and forth to soak up the liquid.

"You couldn't do this over the sink could you?" she yelled.

"You're going to have to go to the hospital," said Tony.

Father and son did not return from the emergency room until two the next morning. Luckily for all of them it was a Saturday. Instead of taking a cab, Tony insisted they walk home. In the pitch black of that cool spring evening, Charlie managed to keep up with his dad's quick pace. When the pair arrived home his mother had coffee ready.

"Why don't you have a cup?" Tony asked Charles.

With those words from his father, a love affair with coffee was born. With that first cup, Charles was hooked.

Later that morning after only a few hours of sleep, Charles played up his injury when he and his father went to visit Nonna. Instead of going through the front door, they entered by way of the dirt driveway that stretched the length of his grandparent's block and allowed residents to pull up behind their homes. As children, they played a lot in the driveway. Sometimes it would be a game of catch and sometimes a race. The driveway bordered the homes on Thirty-sixth Street and Thirty-seventh Street across the street from Charles' house. He and his sister would often walk the length trying to see if they could see their friends.

Charles opened the eight-foot silver iron gate and walked down the narrow concrete path between the neatly planted rows of dirt. The battleship gray basement door, more of a hatch door really, was propped open and leaning against the side of the steps leading to the kitchen. His left hand ran across the door as he stepped down the wide stairs into the basement.

He practiced his best sad face before entering the doorway. He found Nonna by the white stove. The appliance shone in the morning sun accenting the black knobs and trim. Nonna did a double take when she saw Charles's bandaged hand.

"Ciali!" she exclaimed. "Sitta down, what happena?"

The white gauze ran from the middle of his fingers to his wrist. Charles' face was downcast and he pouted a bit as Nonna doted on him. (What's scary is how his daughter, many many years later, would use the same face to get sympathy and lots of attention from her grandparents.)

"Tony?" Nonna looked inquisitively at her son asking what had happened to her grandson.

Tony removed his brown fabric windbreaker as he explained in Italian how Charlie had cut his hand.

"E niente." Tony told his mother it was nothing, nothing serious. But to her it was. Her grandson had been hurt. She quickly guided Charles to the couch and puffed up the pillows for him to lie down. Charles loved the attention.

◆   ◆   ◆

In the cool of the basement they watched the broadcast of the pope's wake on the small eighteen-inch screen. Nonna grabbed her gold-rimmed glasses and joined Josephine on the couch. Charles sat facing them from his seat at the dining table turning his head left to watch the set.

Raised to eye level on a stage of flowers and black cloth, the pope dressed in white and red robes and miter, was protected by blue and yellow uniformed Swiss guards as mourners passed on each side of the body.

"You be il Papa?" Nonna smirked, as she asked her eldest grandchild if he would ever be Pope.

She didn't sound like she was joking. Her eyes glimmered behind the lenses of her gold-rimmed glasses and caught a bit of sunlight as she looked in his direction. While he would have done anything to make his grandmother happy, this was not something he wanted.

"Oh Nonna, I don't think so," Charles laughingly responded. And he meant it.

◆   ◆   ◆

"Is there more than this, do you think? When I'm gone, will there only be a small envelope for someone to sift through?" I asked myself as I thought of my grandparent's lives reduced to this single envelope. There was no making sense of it and my self-questioning only served to add to the throbbing pain in my head as if a thousand jackhammers were on the inside trying to bore a hole through my skull.

"Am I destined to be like them?" The dull roar of a 747 on its final approach to JFK whined past, a good two thousand feet above me, descending to the runway ten miles to the south.

"Once my life is over, will it be able to fit in a small envelope? Is that what I want? Is that my destiny?"

I was angry with myself for hating my life, although at the same time realizing how lucky I was. My desire to always want to be somebody was strong. I didn't want this life of ordinary obscurity, and I did everything to try to change it and spent an even greater amount of time thinking of ways to change it.

"If I only had…" was how I thought I could overcome whatever feelings I was having. I thought if only I had 'it'—whatever 'it' happened to be at that moment—the having would somehow fix everything and rid me of this empty feeling.

I thought, and quite incorrectly, that the 'its' would provide me the validation that I was someone. But every purchase, every dollar spent, did nothing to help how I felt and actually made me feel worse. I knew this.

But where did this all stem? Why was I feeling this way? I felt if I could just get to the heart of the matter and figure out what was causing me to feel this need to change, to be somebody, I could finally conquer my unhappiness.

My mind never stopped thinking. Whether related to a project at the house or at work, my brain was constantly churning, never turning off. Constant thinking was a protective mechanism against my self-inflicted feelings of emptiness.

I flipped the empty envelope containing my grandparent's life onto the brightly colored tablecloth covering the white vinyl patio table. I hated this table and its ordinary nature. It was so bourgeoisie and disgustingly suburban.

With the sky turning a cool shade of periwinkle, I sat in the coolness of the late afternoon, the papers strewn about the table before me still trying to make sense of everything.

19

It's Good to Look Back Every Now and Then

I turned the key, the lock creaked. The storm door rested on my backside as I opened the wooden door. The familiar smell and view greeted me. This time, however, there was no Nonna. Countless times in my life I had stood here like today and waited for the one person who could brighten my day to open the door for me.

My heart grew heavy as I walked through the house one last time. But not alone, my daughter joined me. She would never know her great-grandmother, the woman who brought so much love to this home.

Emptied of its contents, it seemed much more open and spacious, but not as big as it had seemed when I was a kid. I was all at once comforted and depressed. I had spent years trying to find a place that held the same importance for me as this home, but with no luck. Even my own home for all its comfort and aesthetic beauty could not replace what I had been missing from my experiences in this small, two-story dwelling. This was the place I was looking for in my life, the center of what made sense to me. I felt at home.

I walked the length of the hallway looking past the shiny brown tops of my laced oxfords to the floor below. The linoleum's geometric squares with rich browns, beige and a dose of black (used mostly as an outline) had not been replaced for as long as I could remember. The color was patchy and worn in some areas, showing its history.

I walked on the same floor my grandmother had walked. There was a deep sense of history here for me. I moved slowly trying to retrace the steps she had taken all those years ago.

Continuing through the long corridor bridging the entryway to the backyard door, my eyes scanned each crevice and bump on the walls. There were so many days I followed my grandmother along this very path after she opened the front door for me. I was forced on such occasions to slow my usually brisk stride (a trait I developed from having to keep up with my fast walking father) to a gingerly walk, carefully planning my next step so as not to overtake Nonna. This was painful for me, yet even more painful, was the reason I had to do it.

I made it to the kitchen and leaned up against the stark beige walls. As a child I had spent so many evenings in this one little room, and now here I was an adult. My own child, who by this time was roaming fearlessly from one room to the other, peered at me every now and again to 'boo' her dad.

Gabriella was oblivious to the emotional strings that bound me to this home; to the shadows of family dinners, celebrations, and the inevitable demise of all that happiness.

"God, it seems like so long ago," I thought to myself. "Like another lifetime."

It was another lifetime. So many years had passed. I wasn't that same person. But deep down inside, this place represented who I was and helped create who I would be.

Allowing a long audible sigh escape my lips, the heaviness in my chest became more acute.

Gabriella had just made her way through the French doors of the living room and was now exiting what was once her great grandparent's bedroom to join me. She looked at me in the only way she could—innocently. Her brown eyes looked up through strands of shiny auburn hair caressing her forehead.

When I caught her glance she squinted as if I had done something wrong. Or perhaps it was due to the beams of sun coming in through the kitchen window casting cool white rays on the left side of her face.

There were many things time had not changed, like the sun that bathed the rooms much the same way it did back then. Only now, as opposed to bringing a lighthearted feeling, it seemed to accentuate the cracks in the wall, the black chip in the paint of the white kitchen cabinets. All the imperfections of age and neglect were now clearly visible.

Ten months had passed since my grandfather's death. With his affairs finally in order, it had been decided to sell the house. I wanted this one last chance to walk through it. Standing in the kitchen I stared through the window of the silver storm door. I took one long, last glance at the stoop knowing I would never again have the privilege of sitting there talking with my family, with Nonna.

Boom!

I closed the door. It gave me a hard time, almost as if it did not want to close. The lock needed a bit of convincing and a lot of elbow grease before it would latch shut.

"Come on Gab," I whispered to my daughter, a mixture of sadness and a greater sense of finality in my voice. I tried hard not to talk that much due to the huge lump in my throat, now worsening from holding back tears.

Close to twenty years had passed since Nonna had died. For me and indeed the rest of the family, the house was never really the same after that. From then on, I could count on two hands the number of times I had visited the house. Nonno had made changes, rented the basement, and let's not forget got remarried. Along with this new woman, came all new furniture.

The place was always crowded. It was difficult for me to visit after Nonna's death, perhaps because this house became just that, a house. It was no longer the home I knew and loved. It had long lacked that welcoming feeling.

Like my many memories, the space has grown cluttered with the belongings of a new wife. I despised the fact that I couldn't even move about without bumping into a chair or a table when I did decide to visit.

Even the backyard was not free from change. Much like the inside of the house, the yard had grown cluttered with a lot of unnecessary items. Nonno had been so protective of his figs in the last year of his life; he put bells on the branches, so his next-door neighbors and his own in-laws wouldn't try to pick them.

Soon after Nonna passed away, he bought a car and actually started to drive. To house the car, he had built a monstrosity of a garage, a homemade creation of bricks, sheet metal, and two by fours—the exterior painted battleship gray. The same gray that was used on the cellar stairs and door.

I questioned, why in the golden years of his life had he chosen to live like this? He should have also kept the basement and not bothered to rent it out. All these changes over the past years should have prepared me well for today. But still, I found it very difficult for me to walk through the rooms and backyard where I had spent so many of my childhood days.

Although I was depressed the house was being sold, it was at long last, closure for me. I could now go on knowing that everything would be moving on, that finally the other woman would be out of the house once and for all.

"Dad, what's wrong?" my daughter asked, genuinely concerned.

"Nothing Gab," I replied. "Dad's just a little sad."

"Don't worry Dad, I make you feel better," she patted my hand. Her sincerity came through with every word.

I bent down on my left knee and looked into her big brown eyes. "I'm sure you will," I chuckled, placing my left hand on her shoulder. The feel of her cotton blue gingham jacket was soft to the touch.

We walked hand in hand down the tiny corridor from the kitchen to the front door. I stretched out my left hand allowing my palm to touch the walls of the hallway. Despite their age, they still looked freshly painted in the semi-gloss beige paint.

In her final months, Nonna had used this wall so many times as her crutch. Despite her increased difficulty in walking, there were moments, little windows or patches of opportunity, where for a day or two her body permitted her some normalcy, allowing her to actually move about without the use of the walker.

These moments, however, were excruciatingly brief and only gave her and me (who was the only one there for the most part to witness these little miracles), a false sense of hope that the inevitable, by some divine intercession or providence, would pass.

I stopped and placed my right hand at a point on the wall where Nonna would have been able to reach and touch. As I stood facing this spot, my hand perfectly flat against the semi-rough surface of the plaster, I cried wishing that summer hadn't ended the way it did.

◆   ◆   ◆

Charles had been sitting in the living room idly watching television when he heard Nonna's steps coming down the hall. Her black-heeled shoes were making their way from the kitchen to the doors across from where he sat on the gilded couch. The steps were slow and deliberate. As Nonna got closer, her grandson got up and looked at her. Her left arm was holding the wall, her other arm relaxed at her side; brushing lightly against the brown sleeveless dress she wore.

"I do good?" Nonna asked, looking at her grandson for approval. This was the first time in a number of weeks she was able to walk unassisted.

"Wow, Nonna, really good!" he replied.

She was so uplifted.

They wanted things to get better and for a brief moment that June day in 1981, they thought it might.

◆   ◆   ◆

Passing through the double French doors leading to the living room on my right, I glanced up. My eyes swept the room. On the cream-colored walls were the dull etched outlines where pictures had hung. The wall paint, that had been protected from the sun and elements by the backing of the picture, shined a bit brighter and seemed still fresh and young.

Glancing over to the wall directly opposite the double French doors where the sofa once was, the longest of these aged outlines showed just five feet from the floor. The space had once been home to a rectangular landscape photo. It was beautifully done, a chalet and small village. "Perhaps the Alps," I pondered. Enclosing the three-foot by two-foot photo was the most exquisite frame in the house, which was made of a mosaic, a triangular cobalt blue and clear-mirrored glass that complimented the greenery of the trees in the picture.

The nails that had supported the picture protruded a mere half-inch from the wall, painted over in the same ecru, semi-gloss paint. There was nothing to support now. They had earned their rest.

Looking around, I saw the shadows of years past, glimpses of the moments that I had experienced in this room such as Nonna dancing and pouring champagne on New Year's Eve as I and my siblings watched Guy Lombardo perform auld lang syne. It was another New Year's celebration spent at Nonna's while my parents went out. I never minded one bit.

I glanced at the wall to the right of French doors. The three nails that Nonna and I had placed twenty years earlier were still there. My memories of that day are still so lucid.

Nonna and I had gone to a hardware store on Steinway Street to purchase not only the nails, but also some inexpensive frames in which to hang each of her children's wedding photos.

Since it was the holiday season, she asked my opinion about a box of glass ornaments, which I approved of. Besides hanging the photos, we were also planning on pulling the Christmas tree from storage and decorating it that afternoon. I smiled remembering the details of our coming home from our jaunt late that morning and deciding where to place the wedding pictures on the wall above the stereo. Nonna wanted to place them straight across. I suggested placing them diagonally; oldest child, my dad, at the top left, followed by Uncle Diego's in the middle, and Josephine's, the most recent having been married just that year, on the bottom right. Nonna liked my idea and that's what we went with.

Now my fingertips reached for the nails. I touched each one. It was such a simple project, but it was so much more than that for me. The lump in my throat was growing.

I looked at the window in the front room. That room at one time, while Josephine still lived here, had been her bedroom. It was converted to a dining room after she married and moved out.

With a thousand thoughts swirling through my mind, I remembered the decorations Nonna placed on those windows every Christmas; the Nativity beautifully depicted on a fourteen by fourteen inch piece of very thin laminated plastic decorating the center window.

Behind it on the ledge of the inside windowsill had stood a three-candle lamp with orange bulbs giving the window a soothing, spiritual glow on those crisp chilly nights when I went outside and looked back toward the house.

Turning around to my right I saw the corner where the tall and very skinny Christmas tree stood each year. I remembered the boxes of fragile, ornately colored ornaments we placed on the tree.

Gab was singing to herself, her hands behind her back as she leaned against the glass panes of the French door.

"Gab get off that door!" I shouted softly, afraid the glass would break. I walked over and guided her backside off the panes.

Reaching for her hand, we continued to the front door and stepped outside to the landing. I turned around and let the wrought iron storm door, my looking glass into the first floor, lean up against my right shoulder blade. I stopped for one minute and thought I saw Nonna sitting at the far end of the hall waiting for me at the kitchen table. I thought of all those times I had stood in this very spot waiting for her to come open the door and greet me; always ready with a hug and kiss.

I had spent so many years looking for a place that provided me with the same joy that this house once did. I looked for someone who would be there for me no matter what, ready to lend advice and support me. No place and nobody was ever able to replicate the calming feeling I felt here. This little patch of twenty-five by one hundred feet was my oasis, my sanctuary.

Tears streamed down my cheeks and dropped off my chin to the landing.

I closed the thick, wooden front door one final time and swallowed hard, adding more pressure to my already heavy chest. The storm door automatically closed behind me.

Gabriella, having just taken a seat on the top step of the landing, got up and took my hand. We headed down the stairs together, my left hand clasping her right. With my right hand I touched the iron railing. I thought of the many times Nonna touched that railing both when she was well and when she was ill.

There were all those doctor visits; Nonna holding onto the rail while I supported her on the left, placing my body under her left shoulder to take her weight. Unlike my grandmother, the gate had withstood the test of time and was still as sturdy now as then; a different color though. The black changed to a shade of mauve, painted by Nonno just a few years ago.

Gabriella and I had made it to the bottom of the stairs. I quickly opened the gate before us and closed it behind us. I glanced up at the house on this perfect spring day. The air was cool and sweet against my face. I took in a deep breath and let out another audible sigh and stood at the gate for a moment, my hands gripping the cold iron.

My thoughts turned to Gab and my youngest child, Anthony, now only one month old. He would never come to know this house as I did. Anthony was born nine months after Nonno died. Having a son was strange for me, especially after losing Nonno. But I felt that through the name, Anthony Charles, the family name would continue. The week before his birth, I had felt both Nonno's and Nonna's strong presence.

The day of Anthony's birth as I sat outside the operating room, Lisa prepped for the C-section, I felt their presence. There was an overwhelming, totally enveloping sense they were preparing a party. I felt a strong sense of celebration, that there, on the other side, they were commemorating the birth of my son. My stomach sank as if I had taken a free fall off a tall building knowing his great-grand parents would never have a chance to see him, but comforted by the fact of what I experienced the day of his birth.

In the distance, I heard the faint whine of engines. Taking another draught of the cool, invigorating spring air, I looked up in plenty of time to see a plane streaking by. Its silver fuselage caught the sun, reflecting it for an instant before gently fading behind the top edge of the house. It left behind two streaks of white puffiness in the crisp blue sky. When I was young, sitting on Nonna's backyard stoop, I would enjoy watching those planes fly by far up in the sky. I always wished I were on them traveling to some foreign and exotic destination. Their sleek silhouettes were romantic and at the same time powerful.

"Come on Dad," my daughter said insistently. She had grown impatient and pulled on my hand.

Turning away from the house we walked. Glancing back over my right shoulder, I wanted to look at the house that held so many memories; memories that seemed distant, but still so very near to my heart. They all came rushing back like a crashing wave over a rocky coast; making pasta in the basement with Nonna, the Sunday visits with coffee in the front room, those warm spring and summer evenings sitting on the backyard stoop.

There were the sleepovers with my brother, sister and cousins when our parents attended a wedding. The following Sunday morning after Nonna woke us up, she would prepare breakfast.

Most of the sleepovers were just me, spending the night to help Nonna prepare for a holiday meal or just for the heck of it. There were the evenings when Nonna sat side by side on the living room sofa watching *Lawrence Welk* or *The Love Boat* or perhaps *Laverne & Shirley*.

The tears were flowing freely now, tickling the tip of my nose as they glided off and down to the pavement barely missing the tip of my shoe.

"God," I thought. "All these memories seem like a lifetime ago." Actually, I stopped to think, twenty years *is* practically another lifetime.

I was a man now, not some teenager. Married, dealing with the everyday issues and problems that arise in one's life, and blessed with a beautiful daughter and son my grandmother would have adored, and I was sure the feeling would have been mutual.

My introspection was broken with Gab's persistent tugs on my hand. I glanced down. She looked up squinting her eyes from the sun's rays, which by now was setting behind the homes across the street. I gave in to the yanking on my hand and started walking up the block.

My nose burned from the tears which I tried my hardest to suppress. I had walked up this block so many times during my life, sometimes by myself, sometimes with Nonna, at other times with my family. Now here I was, with my daughter.

I momentarily looked to her just as a tiny leaf landed on her head. It didn't stay for long thanks to the gentle breeze that came and whisked it to the sidewalk. She turned her head looking back at the house.

"I can't believe how much like me you are," I said, almost laughing. The collar of my black leather jacket brushed my face. Gabriella was the spitting image of me in terms of looks and attitude and mannerisms, like turning her head back when she walked.

I had done this so much whenever I walked with Nonna, like when I accompanied her to pick Josephine up from work at the bakery. She constantly nudged me, lovingly of course, to stop.

As I walked with Gabriella, I strained my ear hoping I would perhaps hear my grandmother in her broken English telling me, "No turnna around." Unfortunately, time has dealt me a cruel blow and softened my memory of her voice.

Gabriella turned around once more and I was now in the same role that Nonna once was. As I thought to nudge Gab to turn around, I stopped myself.

My hand was inches away from the back of her head. Instead, I patted her shiny auburn hair as we continued to walk the four hundred and ten steps back to my parent's house.

The breeze caressed my face. I realized how truly lucky I was to have known Nonna. Hearing her laugh, seeing her smile, knowing her deep faith, and at the end, understanding the strength of her courage in facing such a brutal illness, made my ordinary life a lot more special.

"You know what?" I thought to myself taking in a deep breath of cool air. "It's good to look back every now and then."

End

978-0-595-38620-8
0-595-38620-2